T0209941

Telemedicine and Asthma:
An innovative approach to
improve morbidity
and mortality rates for
active adults.

Effects of Telemedicine in Asthma care for
remote and inner-city underserved populations.

Musue Kaneh, DHSc, MSN, FNP-C

WESTBOW
P R E S S®
A DIVISION OF THOMAS NELSON
& ZONDERVAN

WestBow Press books may be ordered through booksellers or by contacting:

WestBow Press
A Division of Thomas Nelson & Zondervan
1663 Liberty Drive
Bloomington, IN 47403
www.westbowpress.com
844-714-3454

ISBN: 979-8-3850-1036-3 (sc)
ISBN: 979-8-3850-1037-0 (hc)
ISBN: 979-8-3850-1038-7 (e)

Library of Congress Control Number: 2023920304

Print information available on the last page.

WestBow Press rev. date: 11/01/2023

I thank Diana Willeman-Buckelew, PhD, Milena Staykova, EdD, FNP-C. BC, Judy Jenks, DNP, FNP-BC, and Jeannine Everhart, PhD, of Radford University, Virginia. For their unwavering support and scholarly guidance during the systematic research project endeavor that led to the book's production.

TABLE OF CONTENTS

Abstract   xiii

Chapter 1: Background   1
- ▸ The Impact of Telemedicine in Global Asthma Care   3
- ▸ Statement of the Problem   4
- ▸ The Purpose of the Research Project and the Research Questions   5

Chapter 2: Literature Review   9
- ▸ Telehealth and Telemedicine as Health Care Alternatives   10
- ▸ Impact of Telemedicine on Health Care in the United States   12
- ▸ Telemedicine's Role in Revolutionizing Health Care   13
- ▸ Effects of Telemedicine on Health Care Delivery and
     Quality of Life in Rural and Urban Areas   14
- ▸ Demographics and Barriers Regarding the Use of Telehealth   17
- ▸ Negatives Aspects of and Barriers to Telehealth   20
- ▸ Barriers to Telehealth Adaptation in Rural Areas and
     Communities   22
- ▸ Asthma Treatment, Morbidity, and Mortality   23
- ▸ The Global Burden and Social Effects of Asthma   24
- ▸ Morbidity and Prevalence of Asthma in the United States   25
- ▸ Mortality and Expenses Associated with Asthma in the
     United States   27
- ▸ Standard Treatment of Asthma   27
- ▸ Asthma-related Community Care   28
- ▸ Current Treatment of Asthma   29
- ▸ Disparities in Asthma Care in Urban Regions   30
- ▸ Asthma and Telemedicine in Underserved Populations   31
- ▸ Chapter Summary   33

Chapter 3: Methodology

Chapter 3: Methodology ... 35

▸ Study Design ... 36
▸ Types of Studies for Inclusion and Exclusion ... 37
▸ Data Collection ... 37
▸ Data Analysis ... 40
▸ Limitations ... 44
▸ Delimitations ... 45
▸ Project Summary ... 45

Chapter 4: Results

Chapter 4: Results ... 47

▸ Results ... 47
▸ Excluded Studies ... 56
▸ Effectiveness Measures Due to Telemedicine ... 56
▸ Outcome Measures Due to Telemedicine ... 56
▸ Study Findings Related to Research Questions ... 57
▸ Biases and Limitations of Included Studies ... 62
▸ Summary of Systematic Literature Review Findings ... 63

Chapter 5: Discussion

Chapter 5: Discussion ... 67

Conclusions ... 73
References ... 75
Appendices ... 87

LIST OF FIGURES

Figure 1:   Annual Cases of Deaths Due to Asthma,
            2001 through 2016   2

Figure 2:   Percentages of Adults with Asthma in the
            United States, 2017–2018   3

Figure 3:   United States' Global Outsourcing
            Telemedicine Market Insight, 2019–2025   12

Figure 4:   Telehealth Usage and Willingness in the
            United States, According to Age   17

Figure 5:   Geographic Distribution of Telehealth
            Consumers in the United States   19

Figure 6:   Global Prevalence of Asthma   25

Figure 7:   Self-reported Lifetime of Adult Asthma
            Prevalence (%) According to State or
            Territory in the United States, 2017   26

Figure 8:   Process and Flow of the Systematic
            Literature Review in the Current Project   39

Figure 9:   Selection and Exclusion of Articles for the
            Systematic Literature Review   48

LIST OF TABLES

Table 1: Databases, Keywords, and Phrases Used to
          Identify Articles for Review   38

Table 2: Data Extraction Table   43

Table 3: Kappa Analysis for the Five Studies
          Included for Review   49

Table 4: Kappa Analysis for the Six Excluded Studies   50

LIST OF APPENDICES

Appendix 1: Coding Guidelines   87

Appendix 2: Interpretation of Cohen's Kappa   89

Appendix 3: Selection of the Five Studies to Include
for Review According to the Two Raters   90

Appendix 4: Selection of the Six Studies to Exclude
from Review According to the Two Raters   92

Appendix 5: Data Analysis Table for the Five Articles
in the Systematic Review   94

ABSTRACT

By increasing the quality, accessibility, and efficiency of health care, telemedicine has improved health outcomes worldwide, including those for adults with asthma in the United States. However, access to and utilization of telemedicine by asthmatic adults (18 to 55 years) in poor, inner-city areas are low. This systematic review sought to clarify the impact of telemedicine on asthma morbidity and mortality for inner-city, underserved adults. Six medical databases were searched for literature published between January 1, 2013, and May 31, 2021. The keyword search and systematic review followed PRISMA guidelines; articles for inclusion in the review were assessed independently by two raters. The high inter-rater correlation ($\kappa = 1.0$) indicates the validity of the review process. Of the five studies included in the final analysis, two reported effectiveness measures associated with the use of telemedicine, including significantly decreased acute asthma symptoms, improved medication compliance, and tobacco cessation according to the Asthma Control Test (ACT; $p = 0.005$ for all measures). In addition, more of the patients who participated in telemedicine interventions (49%) achieved a well-controlled asthma score (ACT score >19) than did those in the control group (27%; $p < 0.05$). The remaining three studies in the review focused on adult outcomes, including reduced asthma symptoms, improved quality of life, and decreased morbidity and mortality. Compared with face-to-face asthma care, telemedicine promoted significantly improved outcomes among participating patients, indicated as increased asthma quality of life (0.37; 95% confidence interval, 0.14–0.61) and asthma control (95% confidence interval, 00.26–0.88). The evidence disclosed through this systematic review supports the long-term effectiveness of telemedicine in inner-city, underserved adults with asthma. The study results highlight the need to promote the application of telemedicine for asthma care in underserved areas, given its positive effects on quality of life, morbidity, and mortality.

1

BACKGROUND

Asthma is a global healthcare problem that affects people of all backgrounds and ages. In 2016, there were 339 million cases of asthma worldwide, among which approximately 420,000 people died due to their disease (Center for Disease Control and Prevention [CDC], 2017; World Health Organization [WHO], 2020). The number of cases of asthma worldwide is projected to increase to approximately 400 million by 2025, as countries become more urbanized (To et al., 2012; WHO, 2020). These staggering statistics demonstrate that asthma poses significant risks to the health and quality of life of the global population.

In the United States, asthma accounts for approximately 1.8 million emergency room visits each year, and almost 189,000 people annually receive inpatient treatment because of exacerbation of asthma symptoms (CDC, 2019). More than 25 million people in the United States—approximately one in 13—have asthma. Skillful evaluation and effective control measures are urgently needed to mitigate the severe long-term effects, improve the health outcomes, and reduce the economic burdens associated with asthma.

Despite significant improvements in the diagnosis and treatment of asthma during 2001 through 2016 in the United States, the number and rate of deaths due to the disease have remained stable during this same period (Figure 1) (CDC, 2017). The number of asthma deaths annually in the United States reached the record high of 4,269 in 2001, compared with the data of 3,518 in 2016 (CDC, 2017). Approximately 10 adult American asthmatics died each day (3,564 overall) in 2017 (CDC, 2018).

Figure 1

Annual Cases of Deaths Due to Asthma, 2001 through 2016

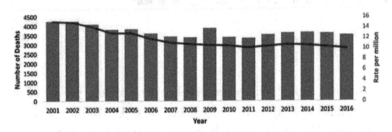

Note: Despite marked advances in evaluation and treatment, deaths due to asthma have not decreased proportionately. Retrieved from https://www.cdc.gov/asthma/asthma_stats/asthma_underlying_death.html.

Compared with their male peers, adult women are five times more likely to die from asthma (American Lung Association [ALA], 2017), particularly African American women, who accounted for approximately 12% of all adult asthma deaths in the United States during 2017 and 2018 (Figure 2) (CDC, 2020). Essentially, 61% of asthma deaths are among women, making the death rate 32% higher among women than men (ALA, 2017). In addition to gender, various racial and ethnic factors are highly associated with asthma frequency and death. Illness and death from asthma positively correlate with poverty, poor urban air quality, indoor allergens, insufficient patient education, and limited access to health care (John et al., 2017).

Figure 2

Percentages of Adults with Asthma in the United States, 2017–2018

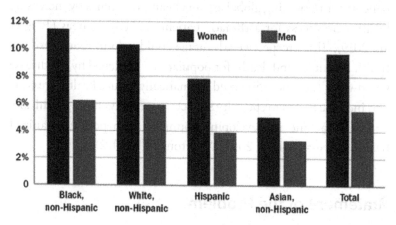

Note. The data in the figure demonstrate the large numbers of adults with asthma, which are highest among Black Americans, despite relevant improvement in diagnostic measures and applied treatment interventions. Retrieved from https://www.mdedge.com/chestphysician/article/224553/asthma/black-women-highest-risk-asthma.

The Impact of Telemedicine in Global Asthma Care

Telemedicine is a subset of telehealth that provides clinical medical services to patients remotely by using technology (American Academy of Family Physicians [AAFP], 2021). WHO (2019) describes telemedicine as a health care delivery service to overcome situations where distance is a limiting factor. Telemedicine assists health care professionals by enabling them to exchange valid information to diagnose, treat, and prevent diseases and injuries; perform research and evaluation; and participate in continuing education events, with the result of enhancing the health of individual people and their communities. Studies of telemedicine have identified its potential benefits for improving global asthma health outcomes by increasing health care access for asthmatic patients in remote areas (Jong et al., 2019). This prospective advantage could help to reduce asthma health inequities and deaths for populations burdened by the disease worldwide. These benefits could dramatically reduce healthcare costs and increase access to specialty services, especially in geographically remote areas and in developing countries with poorly organized health systems (WHO, 2012; Wootton et al., 2012).

Statement of the Problem

Although a preventable disease in many ways, asthma persists. With an incidence rate of 1 in 13 people, affecting approximately 7.7% of American adults and 8.4% of American children (CDC, 2019), asthma affects people of all backgrounds and ages. Approximately 22% of underserved inner-city populations with marginal education and poor access to health care are affected by asthma— often disproportionately (Gergen & Togias, 2015). Despite vigorous improvement in diagnostic and treatment measures, the number of asthma cases continue to rise worldwide and in the United States, especially among indigenous, rural, and poor underserved inner-city populations (CDC, 2020; Jong et al., 2019). These increased case numbers are compounded by limited access to care (CDC, 2020; Leath et al., 2018). As the accessibility and affordability of technological solutions as avenues for communicating with healthcare providers increase, the availability of health care will increase as well.

In 2018, almost 3,500 people died from asthma-related complications (CDC, 2018), and per-person medical costs associated with asthma amounted to nearly $3,300 annually in 2015 (Nurmagambetov et al., 2018). In addition, approximately

10 Americans die from asthma every day (CDC, 2018). Annual asthma-associated costs in the United States are increasing rapidly and steadily, from $12 billion in 1994 to $56 billion in 2011, and are estimated to continue as such (John et al., 2017; Nunes et al., 2017). Asthma therefore presents considerable health and economic burdens to patients, their families, communities, and the government (CDC, 2017; Nunes et al., 2017).

Telemedicine might be an effective alternative for people without means of transportation or who would otherwise have difficulty in obtaining in-person medical care. In particular, whether the inclusion of telemedicine into the health care of people residing in underserved inner-city communities reduces the incidence of adult asthma outbreaks and deaths needs to be understood. By assessing the literature on telemedicine interventions and their effects on asthma care, this systematic review will help to clarify whether telemedicine is an effective strategy for improving the long-term health outcomes of asthmatic patients from underserved populations. Furthermore, it is also important to determine whether telemedicine is an effective way to help patients self-manage their asthma and whether the inclusion of telemedicine in care plans increases patient satisfaction. Investigating these factors will help practitioners develop more effective telemedicine interventions for communities that are disproportionately affected by asthma.

The Purpose of the Research Project and the Research Questions

The purpose of this project was to conduct a systematic review of scientific literature published between January 1, 2013, and May 31, 2021, regarding the influence of telemedicine applications on the long-term health benefits, asthma self-management education, and patient satisfaction of inner-city, underserved adults (18 to 55 years old) who have asthma. Although other systematic reviews involving asthmatic adults have been published (Wainwright & Wootton, 2003; Zhao et al., 2015), they mostly focus on the effectiveness of telemedicine at controlling asthma symptoms rather than on the long-term health benefits that telemedicine can yield. In addition, no published systematic review has explicitly addressed the impacts of telemedicine on underserved adult populations. Given that people from minority and underserved populations tend to suffer disproportionately from asthma (CDC, 2020; John et al., 2017) and from lack of access to health care (Veen et al., 2019), understanding how telemedicine influences the long-term health of asthma patients, as well as morbidity and mortality rates, in these subpopulations is particularly important. Therefore, the main objective of this project was to synthesize the published literature to reveal whether telemedicine improves long-term health outcomes and decreases morbidity and mortality rates in inner-city adult asthmatics. An additional goal was to enhance healthcare practitioners' awareness of the benefits of telemedicine by providing a comprehensive overview of the data regarding the effectiveness of telemedicine and asthma treatment in underserved populations.

This systematic review included studies published between 2013 and 2021 and that used quantitative, qualitative, and mixed-method approaches. The project addressed the following research questions (Q) and associated hoped-for outcomes (O).

> Q1. In underserved inner-city adults (18 to 55 years old) with asthma, what is the effect of telemedicine conferences compared with face-to-face office visits on self-reported quality of life?

> O1. The hoped-for outcome to this question was that the literature review would support higher self-reported quality of life associated with telemedicine

intervention than face-to-face office visits among underserved adults (18 to 55 years old) with asthma.

Q2. Compared with face-to-face treatment, how effective is telemedicine in decreasing asthma morbidity among underserved inner- city adults (18 to 55 years old)?

O2. The hoped-for outcome for this question was that the literature review would support the effectiveness of telemedicine in decreasing asthma morbidity to be equal to or better than face-to-face visits among underserved inner-city adults (18 to 55 years old).

Q3. Compared with face-to-face specialist treatment, how effective is telemedicine in decreasing asthma mortality among underserved inner- city adults (18 to 55 years old)?

O3. The hoped-for outcome for this question was that the literature review would support the effectiveness of telemedicine in decreasing asthma mortality to be equal to or better than face-to-face specialist visits among underserved inner-city adults (18 to 55 years old).

Chapter 1 provides background information for the present project. The contents describe the significance of the study and the important implications of using telemedicine with asthmatic patients. In addition, Chapter 1 outlines the project's purpose and research questions. Chapter 2 provide a synthesis of the literature regarding the use of telemedicine in asthmatic populations.

LITERATURE REVIEW

Research on telemedicine is accumulating. Considerable research that discusses the effects of telemedicine on the healthcare industry is available (Alvandi, 2017; Branning & Vater, 2016; Totten et al., 2020). Evidence regarding the benefits that telemedicine can yield in rural or traditionally underserved communities is noted (Ferrer-Rocio et al., 2010; Leath et al., 2018). One of the most important aspects of telemedicine is that it provides an alternative source of health care to people who, due to transportation or mobility issues, would otherwise have difficulty accessing traditional forms of health care (CDC, 2020).

In addition, telemedicine offers marginalized, inner-city Latino and African American populations attractive advantages including reduced waiting times and increased access (George et al., 2009). The of use telemedicine to help patients with asthma manage and control their symptoms has been studied previously (Chongmelaxme et al., 2019; Erquicia et al., 2016). However, this previous research typically has been conducted in schools (Bian et al., 2019; Perry & Turner, 2019) or rural settings (Perry et al., 2018; Taylor et al., 2019) rather than with underserved inner-city populations. Therefore, the present project will help to fill a gap in the literature regarding the use of telemedicine with inner-city asthmatic adults.

This chapter, Chapter 2, synthesizes the relevant literature regarding the use of telemedicine in asthmatic populations, with a particular focus on the use of telemedicine in underserved communities. The chapter begins with a broad overview of the use of telemedicine and its influence on health care in the United States. The advantages and disadvantages that telemedicine presents to underserved populations, especially rural and minority communities, are then explored; standard treatments are presented; and morbidity and mortality rates in the United States are discussed. Chapter 2 ends with an analysis of previous reviews of the use of telemedicine in treating asthma.

Telehealth and Telemedicine as Health Care Alternatives

Telehealth refers to the use of technology to deliver medical care and treatment in a remote setting (AAFP, 2021). The term telehealth is used to refer to a broad array of clinical and non-clinical services that are provided at a distance, including the diagnosis and treatment of disease, research, monitoring, and continuing education (WHO, 2021). More than half of the 70 member countries of the WHO have a national telehealth policy (WHO, 2021), thus demonstrating that telehealth is a common alternative to conventional face-to-face forms of health care.

Telemedicine is the subset of telehealth that refers to the provision of clinical services at a distance to improve health care delivery through a wide range of applications, with the benefit of improving access to care in all parts of the world (AAFP, 2021; Wootton et al., 2012). Similarly, the Center for Medicare and Medicaid Services (CMS) describes telemedicine as a technology that seeks to improve patients' health through two-way, real-time interactive communication between patients and practitioners at distant sites that is accomplished by their engagement in electronic communication via interactive telecommunications equipment that includes, at minimum, both audio and video elements (CMS, 2020). The practice of telemedicine is estimated to have begun in the 1960s, even though the term 'telemedicine' itself is relatively new (Doorn et al., 2014).

In some countries such as the United States, telemedicine has dramatically reduced health care costs and increased access to specialty services for populations in inner cities and remote rural communities (Jong et al., 2019). Thus, healthcare providers and professionals can utilize advanced information and communication technology through telemedicine services to improve overall health care outcomes in diverse clinical settings (Almathami et al., 2019; Kim & Zuckerman, 2019). This prospective advantage would help to reduce health care inequities and to strengthen health systems in developing countries (WHO, 2012; Wootton et al., 2012).

As a nonmedical example of the increasing use and popularity of telehealth modalities, the global telemedicine market is growing, particularly in developing countries such as China and India (Figure 3). This growth likely reflects the potential benefits of telemedicine in improving global health outcomes through increased health care access, especially for indigenous populations throughout the world; this increased access is a result of the significantly reduced cost of telemedicine compared with traditional modes (Jong et al., 2019). In addition, on the global research agenda, the telemedicine initiative connects medical professionals worldwide (Dinesen et al., 2016). Telemedicine thereby contests against various—sometimes longstanding—political policies, particularly those restricting access to foreign educational resources and limiting international communication. In this context, telemedicine can reduce the harmful effects of such policies on the health care system in countries such as North Korea, thereby demonstrating telemedicine's ability to overcome physical, geopolitical, economic, and social barriers (Dinesen et al., 2016; Mistry, 2012). Telemedicine provides opportunity to mitigate the negative effects of multiple social or political factors.

Figure 3

United States' Global Outsourcing Telemedicine Market Insight, 2019–2025

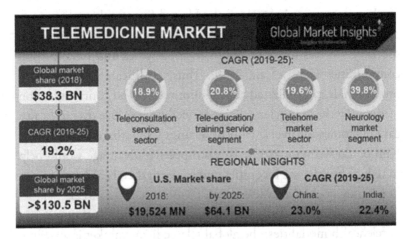

Note. This figure presents the compound annual growth rate (CAGR) percentages of the telemedicine global market insights for China and India during 2019 through 2025 and illustrates the rapid growth of the telemedicine industry globally. Retrieved from https://www.mpo-mag.com/contents/view_online-exclusives.

Impact of Telemedicine on Health Care in the United States

The United States healthcare system is the most expensive globally, with an estimated 3.2 trillion (equivalent to 17.8% of the gross domestic product) spent on healthcare costs in 2015 (Branning & Vater, 2016). In addition, the numbers of both insured and uninsured people who live in inner cities and rural areas with limited access to traditional modes of health care are rising, thus increasing the demand for hospital services, doctors' office visits, and prescription medications (Branning & Vater, 2016). By reducing barriers to care for people with geographic, transportation, or mobility issues, telemedicine can markedly benefit traditionally medically underserved populations (CDC, 2020).

In the United States, the use of telemedicine has expanded exponentially since the late 1990s and was projected to grow into a $30 billion share of the health care market by the end of 2020, with a notable increase of $20.4 billion since 2013 and an anticipated rise of more than $67 billion by 2024 (Bhaskar et al., 2020; CDC, 2020). Increased access to telemedicine services, the recognition of telehealth as a standard of care, telemedicine's positive influence on the provider–patient relationship, and the potential to save billions of dollars in healthcare costs have all contributed to the phenomenal growth of the United States' telemedicine industry (CDC, 2020; Mistry, 2012).

Telemedicine has reduced health care costs and provided increased access to specialty services for inner-city and rural American communities (Jong et al., 2019). However, the rapid, widespread implementation of telemedicine requires careful research of its effects on patient healthcare outcomes.

Telemedicine's Role in Revolutionizing Health Care

One of the aims of telemedicine is to meet the needs of today's healthcare consumers by revolutionizing health care delivery (Alvandi, 2017). Telemedicine supports efforts to improve the quality of health care by increasing accessibility and efficiency to health care by reducing the need to travel, providing clinical support, overcoming geographic barriers, offering various communication mechanisms, and improving patient outcomes. Thus, health care should consider the current focus on efforts to contain costs, improve the delivery of care to all segments of the patient population, and meet consumer demand, telemedicine is an attractive tool (Alvandi, 2017; CDC, 2020). Furthermore, Totten et al. (2020) noted telemedicine's rapid expansion as an indicator of its being both a solution to current problems and an innovation whose time has come. For example, health care in the United States and many other countries transformed rapidly out of the need to respond to the COVID-19 pandemic.

Courageous efforts supported this transformation, which ranged from converting hospital spaces and nonmedical facilities into intensive care units to implementing new clinical guidelines and policies. Perhaps the most evident and wide-reaching of these changes was the telehealth explosion (Totten et al., 2020). At the pandemic's peak, telemedicine utilization provided and supported health care delivery across time and distance, expanded access, facilitated information exchange, and delivered care in alternative formats. Telemedicine applications provided for remote patient monitoring of acute and chronic health conditions, allowing for critical maintenance care at a distance. In addition, telemedicine allowed patients—particularly those in remote areas—to receive care, including psychiatric counseling and other treatments, in the privacy of their homes or alternative locations (Totten et al., 2020). It demonstrated the efficiency of telemedicine in being a dependable source of healthcare for the population in the United States and other parts of the world during a crisis period when an alternative means of healthcare provision was urgently needed.

Effects of Telemedicine on Health Care Delivery and Quality of Life in Rural and Urban Areas

Growing evidence supports telemedicine as a cost-effective and powerful tool with the potential to improve rural health care (CDC,

2020; Leath et al., 2018). Approximately 15% to 20% of Americans (60 million people) live in rural areas (CDC, 2020). Compared with urban and suburban populations, residents of rural areas in the United States face substantial challenges in accessing health care and have overall poorer health outcomes, including higher rates of chronic disease, higher death rates, and delayed diagnoses for cancers and other diseases (CDC, 2020; Leath et al., 2018). In 2017, estimated percentages of potentially preventable deaths from chronic lower-respiratory disease ranged from 13.0 % in urban communities to 57.1% in rural areas (Miller, 2019). This high death rate from chronic respiratory disease demonstrates the devastating effects due to barriers to health care access in rural areas.

Telemedicine improves health care access, which is a continuous challenge for rural communities (Leath et al., 2018). In addition, telemedicine increases rural residents' contact with specialty care providers and decreases the long-distance travel necessitated by the accelerated closure of hospitals and clinic in recent years. Although not a complete solution, telemedicine nonetheless can address many of these issues and, in turn, help to narrow the rural–urban health divide.

A randomized study conducted by Ferrer-Rocio et al. (2010) assessed telemedicine's impact on quality of life among patients living in rural areas. The authors used questionnaires to evaluate the well-being and health status of 800 primary care patients referred for specialized care—420 patients referred to hospitals for traditional face-to-face care and 380 patients referred to hospital specialists through telemedicine. Both groups demonstrated similar improvements in health status. For example, 45 (11.8%) of the 380 patients in the telemedicine group reported that their health status was much better after receiving care, whereas 52 (12.3%) of the 420 patients in the face-to-face group reported feeling much better. Furthermore, 98 patients (25.8%) that participated in telemedicine reported a final pain level of 'low', compared with 100 patients (23.8%) in the face-to-face group.

In summary, the experience and outcomes of patients who

received specialist care via telemedicine were comparable to those who were referred to hospitals for face-to-face medicine. However, a key benefit of telemedicine was that participants in that study group did not have to travel. Consequently diagnoses, examinations, and treatments were initiated more rapidly for telemedicine than for those who received hospital referrals, thus positively influencing the quality of care, quality of life, and treatment outcomes.

Barriers to health care access are not only geographic but ethnic and socioeconomic. One qualitative study (George et al., 2009) involved 10 focus groups of African American and Latino participants (n = 87; African American, n = 43 [49%]; Latino, n = 44 [51%]) in a historically underserved area of inner-city, south-central Los Angeles. The study's purpose was to explore perceptions about the innovative care provided through telemedicine and its potential to increase specialty care access among underserved urban populations. Approximately 33% of parents and seniors had some high-school education, and 33% were high-school graduates. Overall, 25% of both groups had some college education, but more seniors (18%) than parents (10%) were college graduates.

The study's results demonstrated that for both African Americans and Latinos telemedicine offered several advantages as compared with their usual modes of health care. Most of these advantages centered around reduced waiting time, immediate feedback regarding diagnosis and course of treatment plan, and increased access to specialists and to multiple medical opinions as required (George et al., 2009). For these (and other) minority groups, the larger socioeconomic context presents several barriers to health care access and utilization. In particular, the participants, who resided in a socioeconomically disadvantaged community, overwhelmingly identified timely access to care as one of the greatest advantages of telemedicine (George et al., 2009).

Telemedicine provides some relatively quick solutions to challenges involving transportation to specialist care, timely access to specialists, efficient communication, and the need for multiple medical opinions in specialist-scarce zones. The findings from the studies cited above (Ferrer-Rocio et al., 2010; George et al., 2009) support the potential long-term benefits of telemedicine in historically underserved areas in the United States.

Demographics and Barriers Regarding the Use of Telehealth

Relatively little is known regarding how telehealth usage might differ across different demographic groups, geographic location (urban vs. rural), and insurance status. A 2019 survey on telehealth usage in the United States revealed that 66% of consumers were willing to use telehealth, with most of the interest stemming from younger generations (Figure 4) (American Well, 2019). However, approximately half of the seniors who responded were opened to using telehealth, especially for prescription and chronic care management (American Well, 2019).

Figure 4
Telehealth Usage and Willingness in the United States, According to Age

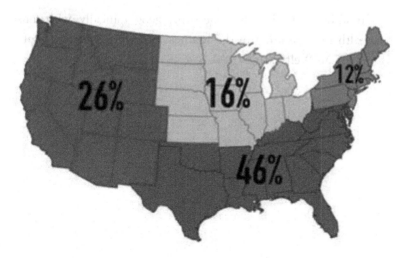

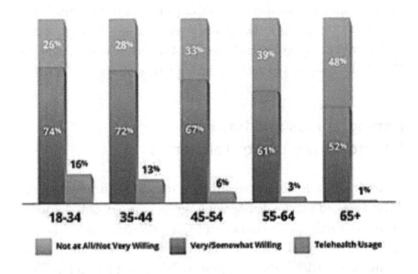

Note: According to survey responses, the predominant users of telehealth were 18 to 34 years old. However, more than half of participants 65 and older were willing to use telehealth modalities, although they did not currently. Retrieved from https://static. americanwell.com/app/uploads/2019/07/American-Well-Telehealth-Index-2019- Consumer-Survey-eBook2.pdf.

In addition, telehealth usage varies geographically, with most telehealth users residing in the southeastern United States (Figure 5) (American Well, 2019).

Figure 5

Geographic Distribution of Telehealth Consumers in the United States

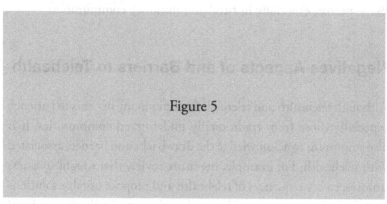

Figure 5

Note: The greatest proportion of users lives in the southeast. Retrieved from https://static.americanwell.com/app/uploads/2019/07/American-Well-Telehealth-Index-2019- Consumer-Survey-eBook2.pdf.

Almost half of all telemedicine users in the United States live in the southeast. In this region of the country, an increased proportion of the population resides in rural areas, where access to conventional health care often is limited. In addition, as will be discussed later, asthma is significantly more prevalent in the southeastern United States than in other regions (CDC, 2017), thus suggesting that telehealth and telemedicine may be helpful alternative health care options for these communities. It is important to recognize that, in addition to differences according to age and geographic region, telehealth use also varies widely by race. A cross-sectional analysis on telehealth usage at the onset of the COVID-19 pandemic revealed that people from minority communities, such as African Americans, and Americans living in rural areas—particularly women and older people—were less likely to have a telehealth visit than people living in urban areas (Pierce & Stevermer, 2020). Indeed, people from rural areas constituted only 20% of telehealth appointments during a 30-day period in 2020, and only 10% of telehealth visits were with

Black or African American patients (Pierce & Stevermer, 2020). These figures suggest that barriers to telehealth and telemedicine usage persist, especially in rural and minority communities.

Negatives Aspects of and Barriers to Telehealth

Although telehealth and telemedicine offer many benefits to patients, especially those from traditionally underserved communities, it is also important to acknowledge the drawbacks and barriers associated with telehealth. For example, literature review that sought to assess unforeseen consequences of telehealth and propose suitable solutions to improve patient care disclosed various technology-associated limitations to the use of telemedicine. Given that the technologic tools for providing telemedicine are continually evolving, patients, families, and healthcare practitioners need continuous education and retraining regarding these tools (Gogia et al., 2016); thus, there is a dual requirement of the evidence-based provision of care. These are effectively addressed by using clinical decision support systems and adaptive learning strategies for all participants (Gogia et al., 2016).

A recent, lengthy systematic literature review investigated the barriers and facilitators that influence home telemedicine consultation systems in the healthcare context (Almathami et al., 2020). The review framework comprised 17 facilitators and 8 barriers, further categorized as internal and external influences, of Home Online Health Consultation (HOHC) systems. Participants in the study ranged from 2 years to older than 80 years with various health problems that could benefit from remote health services, such as controlling chronic respiratory symptoms. The findings showed that HOHC via telehealth conferencing effectively delivered online treatment and—because it simulated in-person, face-to-face consultation—was well-accepted by the participants. In particular, patient acceptance increased because online consultation facilitators promoted effective and convenient remote treatment (Almathami et al., 2020). In contrast to this favorable response, the study's results also demonstrated that some participants preferred face-to-face consultation to online consultancy and were resistant to the online consultation intervention (Almathami et al., 2020).

Several barriers to online consultancy influenced participants' resistance to this intervention. For example, 12 (27%) of the 45 articles used in the systematic review posed concerns regarding potential loss of privacy (Almathami et al., 2020). In addition, lack of knowledge of or unfamiliarity with the system's use were crucial factors for dislike of online consultation (Almathami et al., 2020). 11% of the participants listed lack of knowledge, unfamiliarity with communication technology, and fear of the unknown as leading to resistance to using the HOHC technology; these factors were compounded by insufficient staff training, which hampered effective implementation of online consultation for participants' optimal engagement. Furthermore, approximately 15% to 20% of the participants who had not disclosed their health conditions to their families expressed concern regarding the potential that a family member would overhear their information (Almathami et al., 2020). Another reported concern was that care givers might incidentally see another member of the patient's household during the video-conferencing consultation (Almathami et al., 2020).

Approximately 52% of elderly participants (mean age, 76.75 years) reported that they did not like the lack of physical contact during a telehealth visit and that they might find it challenging to use telemedicine without the assistance of a caretaker or family member (Almathami et al., 2020). However, another segment of the study revealed that, despite their concerns, older patients nonetheless were successful in using telehealth options and did report additional participation difficulties. Therefore, the authors did not consider age to have a significant influence on the use of HOHC (Almathami et al., 2020). Contrary to many preconceptions regarding their potential lack of technology knowledge, older adults are often willing and able to use various forms of telemedicine.

Barriers to Telehealth Adaptation in Rural Areas and Communities

Several barriers to telemedicine in most rural areas, especially rural communities in developing countries, are well recognized. Two of the most frequently noted barriers are the poor-quality cellular networks that serve these regions and poor understanding of how to use the technology necessary for telemedicine (Duclos et al., 2017; Goodridge & Marciniuk, 2016; Sabesan et al., 2018). Data from a sizeable interdisciplinary study listed technology as one of the pivotal barriers in adopting telehealth in rural areas in the United States and other parts of the world (Hampshire et al., 2017).

The most common obstacle in rural areas is the inconsistent cellular network; this inconsistency arises because of the physical distance between rural areas and network towers, which typically are in urban areas. It impacts many rural communities' services to primarily have a limited range that cannot scale to reach a large demographic (Goodridge & Marciniuk, 2016). In addition, many rural residents lack a constant power source to maintain the system, leading to unstable network availability (Duclos et al., 2017; Sabesan et al., 2018).

Significant advances in telehealth technology services in rural communities have been made to overcome technical issues and provide stable access for both patients and providers (Schwamm et al., 2017). For example, problems regarding cellular network inconsistency were alleviated through the distribution of mobile applications to geographically isolated communities, particularly in developing countries, in parts of Europe, and among the indigenous population of rural America. This distribution thereby increased direct connection to mobile devices for healthcare providers' use in local hospitals and clinics (Schwamm et al., 2017).

Another critical barrier to the implementation of telehealth in rural communities in the United States and other parts of the world has been insufficient trained staff for adequate utilization of telehealth programs (Jayasinghe et al. (2016), Liu et al. (2019), Sabesan et al.

(2018), and Taylor et al. (2015). This deficiency has led to limited use of new telehealth equipment and the inability of staff to successfully educate patients in effective telehealth engagement with providers (Jayasinghe et al., 2016; Liu et al., 2019; Sabesan et al., 2018; Taylor et al., 2015). The realization of this drawback prompted of the originators of several telehealth programs to offer classes after hours for health professionals and staff to enhance their understanding and effective use of telehealth systems. In addition, one study's findings supported the incorporation of a telehealth educational incentive as a monetary reward, thus encouraging healthcare providers at all levels to seek continuing education opportunities to improve their proficiency in telehealth technology (Kruse et al., 2018).

Asthma Treatment, Morbidity, and Mortality

Now that the benefits and barriers associated with telemedicine have been explored, an overview of asthma, common treatments of the disease, and the applications of telemedicine in asthma treatment will be presented. Asthma affects approximately 339 million people worldwide and is projected to increase to 400 million by 2025 as countries became more urbanized (To et al., 2012; WHO, 2020). In 2016, an estimated 420,000 people died globally from asthma—more than 100 people daily—with wide rate variations between continents, regions, ages, and economic groups (Asher et al., 2018). The word 'asthma' originates from a Greek word that denotes 'short of breath,' meaning that, initially, any patient with breathlessness was an asthmatic (Holgate, 2010). By the early 1900s, however, the physiologic process of bronchial narrowing due to the constriction of the airway's smooth muscle was experimentally documented and proposed as being a consequence of asthma (Walter & Holtzman, 2015). Quirt et al. (2018) defined asthma as the chronic inflammation associated with airway hyperresponsiveness (i.e., the exaggerated narrowing of airways in response to specific triggers, such as viruses, allergens, and exercise). This hyperresponsiveness leads to recurrent wheezing episodes, breathlessness, chest tightness, and coughing that can vary in duration and intensity (Quirt et al., 2018).

Although various critical environmental determinants that trigger asthma are well-established, more work is needed to define the role of environmental exposures in the development of asthma in both children and adults (Quirt et al., 2018; Walter & Holtzman, 2005). Focusing on the interrelationship between the environment and genetic determinants to identify factors that create high-risk groups and identifying key modifiable exposures could help to decrease improve the morbidity and mortality associated with asthma (Dharmage et al., 2019; Quirt et al., 2018).

The Global Burden and Social Effects of Asthma

The WHO (2020) considers asthma as one of the world's major noncommunicable diseases (Figure 6). WHO (2020) ranked asthma 16th among the leading causes of years lived with disability and 28th among the leading causes of disease burden. Worldwide, the incidence and prevalence of asthma are higher in children, whereas morbidity and mortality are higher in adults and those with severe disease (Dharmage et al., 2019). Asthma is a significant global source of economic burden on individual people, businesses, and governments. In addition to causing patients to accrue more than $3,000 on average in medical expenses annually, asthma is estimated to have caused more than $81.9 billion in losses due to missed work and school days between 2008 and 2013 (Nurmagambetov et al., 2018). Through associated direct and indirect costs, asthma compounds the progressive disability of those affected worldwide, especially those in developing countries, due to limited health resource utilization and poor quality of life (To et al., 2012; WHO, 2020). The financial burdens of asthma are compounded by numerous socioeconomic factors.

Figure 6
Global Prevalence of Asthma

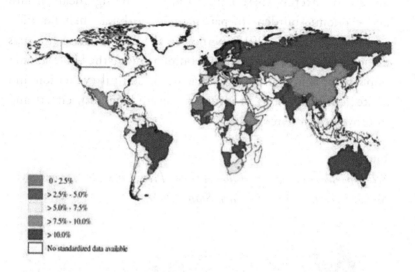

Note. This map shows overall the prevalence of asthma across the world's continents. Asthma is particularly prevalent in Australia, Brazil, and some parts of Europe. Retrieved from www.bmcpublichealth.biomedcentral.com.

Morbidity and Prevalence of Asthma in the United States

More than 25 million people (i.e., approximately one in 13) in the United States have asthma (CDC, 2017). Asthma is more prevalent in the southeastern United State, where disease prevalence exceeds 50% in some states (Figure 7). In 2016, 1.8 million people visited an emergency department for acute asthma-related care, whereas 189,000 people received inpatient treatment because of asthma exacerbation symptoms (CDC, 2017). In addition, an estimated 40 million people in the United States (13% of the population) suffered from asthma lifelong, whereas 26 million (8%) experienced an acute incident of asthma in 2012 (Nunes et al., 2017). Overall, these figures illustrate the significant health and economic burdens to patients with asthma, their families, and society (CDC, 2017; Nunes et al., 2017). These findings demonstrate that asthma's health burden among the United States population is a vital concern that needs skillful evaluation and strategic interventions to minimize severe long-term effects and improve health outcomes.

Figure 7

Self-reported Lifetime of Adult Asthma Prevalence (%) According to State or Territory in the United States, 2017

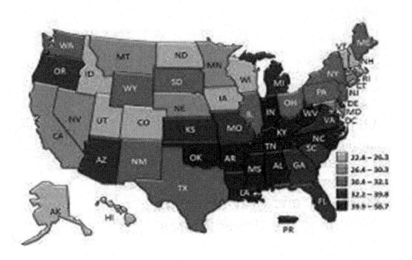

Note. In some southeastern states, asthma prevalence among adults exceeds 50%. Retrieved Date from http://www.cdc.gov/asthma/ surv-reporting.html.

Mortality and Expenses Associated with Asthma in the United States

In 2017, approximately 10 Americans died daily (3,564 total) from asthma (CDC, 2018). Many of these deaths likely could have been avoided with appropriate treatment and supportive care (ALA, 2017; CDC, 2017). Adult women, especially African American women, are at least four times more likely to die from asthma than any other group (CDC, 2017). Illness severity and death due to asthma positively correlate with poverty, low urban air quality, indoor allergens, insufficient patient education, and poor health care (John et al., 2017). As a regional example of asthma mortality, in 2017, Texas experienced 232 deaths related to asthma—equivalent to a death rate of 8.3 per 1 million people (CDC, 2017).

The cost to treat asthma varies from country to country (WHO, 2020). In 2013, the estimated annual economic cost of asthma in the United States was $81.9 billion, representing an average yearly cost of $3,266 per person with the disease (CDC, 2017). In addition, the mean annual personal cost per patient, for all American asthmatics overall, is approximately $1,900 (Nunes et al., 2017). Regardless of a patient's country of residence, asthma is financially burdensome.

Standard Treatment of Asthma

Asthma is the most common respiratory disorder in several regions of the world (WHO, 2020). Despite significant improvement in the diagnosis and management of this disorder, most of the world's population live in regions where asthma remains poorly controlled (CDC, 2017; WHO, 2020). In most asthmatics, optimal control can be achieved by using trigger avoidance and pharmacologic interventions (Quirt et al., 2018). So-called 'relief drugs' are used on an as-needed basis for rapid alleviation of bronchoconstriction and other asthma symptoms (Quirt et al., 2018). In contrast, most used agents for the treatment of asthma are classified as controllers, which are long-term, daily medications that modulate asthma primarily through their anti-inflammatory effects. Controller medications include inhaled corticosteroids, leukotriene receptor antagonists, long-acting beta-agonists in combination with an inhaled corticosteroid, long-acting muscarinic receptor antagonists, and biologic agents including anti-IgE and anti-IL- 5 therapies. In addition, systemic corticosteroid therapy has demonstrated essential efficacy in managing acute asthma exacerbations (Quirt et al., 2018).

Asthma-related Community Care

Community-based approaches to asthma care and treatment are alternative methods to traditional asthma treatments that are delivered by primary care physicians. Common components of community-based interventions include the provision of self-management skills, asthma education, care coordination, and home visits to assess environmental triggers (Holder-Niles et al., 2017; Kennedy et al., 2017; Kercsmar et al., 2017). Community-based interventions are particularly common approaches to the treatment of childhood asthma, with many interventions using schools and home visits to promote self- management education and awareness about different asthma triggers (Chan et al., 2021). Providing asthma education to school staff, improving communication between schools and primary-care providers, and creating asthma-friendly school environments are other community-based approaches to the treatment of asthma in children (Holder-Niles et al., 2017; Naar et al., 2018; Rapp et al., 2018). A systematic review of the effectiveness of community-based interventions on improving asthma outcomes in children found that interventions comprising multiple components and strategies were most successful (Chan et al., 2021). Community-based interventions also have the potential to reduce the economic costs associated with asthma. For example, community-based treatments reduced school absenteeism (Dor et al., 2018); Turyk et al., 2013) and decreased the number of days at work missed by parents due to their child's asthma (Lob et al., 2011).

Asthma is a prevalent disease, both globally and within the United States. With approximately 10 people dying from asthma-related causes daily (CDC, 2018), the disease is a leading cause of preventable deaths in the United States. Globally, asthma is ranked 28th as a leading cause of disease burden, and the disease disproportionately affects populations in developing countries due to poor quality of care and limited access to treatment (To et al., 2012). In the United States, women are more likely than men to die from asthma (CDC, 2017), and minority populations are disproportionately affected due to high poverty levels, poor access to care, and low urban air quality (John et al., 2017). Although an incurable disease, asthma is commonly managed through medications including inhaled corticosteroids and leukotriene receptor antagonists (Quirt et al., 2018). In addition, community-based interventions that promote awareness about asthma triggers, the creation of asthma-friendly environments, and better care coordination can be effective ways of controlling asthma, particularly among children (Holder-Niles et al., 2017; Kennedy et al., 2017). Appropriate management of asthma's symptoms and triggers is key to preventing the development of more serious conditions.

Current Treatment of Asthma

Asthma is the most common respiratory disorder in several regions of the world (WHO, 2020). Despite significant improvement in the diagnosis and management of this disorder, most of the world's population live in regions where asthma remains poorly controlled (CDC, 2017; WHO, 2020). In most asthmatics, optimal control can be achieved by using trigger avoidance and pharmacologic interventions (Quirt et al., 2018). So-called 'relief drugs' are used on an as-needed basis for rapid alleviation of bronchoconstriction and other asthma symptoms (Quirt et al., 2018). In contrast, most used agents for the treatment of asthma are classified as controllers, which are long-term, daily medications that modulate asthma primarily through their anti-inflammatory effects. Controller medications include inhaled corticosteroids, leukotriene receptor antagonists, long-acting beta-agonists in combination with an inhaled corticosteroid, long-acting muscarinic receptor antagonists, and biologic agents including anti-IgE and anti-IL- 5 therapies. In addition, systemic corticosteroid therapy has demonstrated essential efficacy in managing acute asthma exacerbations (Quirt et al., 2018).

Community-based approaches to asthma care and treatment are alternative methods to traditional asthma treatments that are delivered by primary care physicians. Common components of community-based interventions include the provision of self-management skills, asthma education, care coordination, and home visits that assess environmental triggers (Holder-Niles et al., 2017; Kennedy et al., 2017; Kercsmar et al., 2017). Community-based interventions also have the potential to reduce the economic costs associated with asthma. For example, community-based treatments reduced school absenteeism (Dor et al., 2018); Turyk et al., 2013) and decreased the number of days at work missed by parents due to their child's asthma (Lob et al., 2011).

In summary, appropriate management of asthma's symptoms and triggers is key to preventing the development of more serious conditions. Effective treatment of asthma typically involves a multi-faceted approach that combines the avoidance of known triggers, appropriate medications, and patient education in disease self-management.

Disparities in Asthma Care in Urban Regions

Factors such as low socioeconomic status, poverty, and infrastructural inequalities tend to be concentrated in urban areas, particularly among inner-city communities (AAFA, 2020; CDC, 2019). Community health centers often serve as the main drivers to reduce healthcare disparities and provide culturally sensitive services (Childs et al., 2019). However, noteworthy barriers to community-based asthma treatment in urban areas remain, including insufficient primary care physicians and appointments (Childs et al., 2019). For example, in a survey of 395 caregivers, only 23% of patients with asthma conditions had a primary care doctor, whereas 29% frequently visited the emergency room because of their asthma (Sadreameli et al., 2018).

Lack of education decreased access to resources, and Medicare-imposed limits on physician visits are often-cited reasons why people do not have primary care doctors (Kim & Pirration, 2019; Trivedi et al., 2017). In addition, poor air quality in crowded inner-city areas is positively related to asthma symptoms (Kranjac et al., 2017), creating an increased need for treatment. These findings suggest that telemedicine, as a remote-based health care delivery service, may be a viable alternative for inner-city populations who are disproportionately affected by asthma.

Asthma and Telemedicine in Underserved Populations

Little previous research has focused on telemedicine's effects on the care of underserved adults (18 to 55 years old) living with asthma in the United States or elsewhere in the world. Most of the past research focused predominantly on telemedicine's effects on patients' hospital readmissions, quality of life, disease self-management, and symptom control in rural areas. (Chongmelaxme et al., 2019; Erquicia et al., 2016; Lombardi et al., 2015). The contexts and findings of relevant studies are discussed below.

Survey questionnaires were used to evaluate telemedicine's influence on health care demand for patients in Europe with severe, persistent asthma, which was associated with a lack of education about the disease (Erquicia et al., 2016). Participants used a peak flow meter for assessment, with data reported daily through a tablet and reviewed every 2 to 4 weeks during a video conference with a physician to determine whether the current treatment plan was adequate or required adjustment for optimal symptom control. Analysis of the data showed that, through increased patient education, telemedicine led to a 28% decline in hospital admissions, a 90% decline in emergency room visits, improved symptom management, and enhanced quality of life among European asthmatics (Erquicia et al., 2016).

A systematic review and meta-analysis of 22 studies involving 10,281 participants in total revealed that telemedicine—alone or in combination with other approaches and as case-management interventions—improved asthma symptom control and quality of life among adult participants compared with effects achieved through traditional care measures (Chongmelaxme et al., 2019). In addition, a review of 21 randomized controlled trials evaluated the effects of telehealth visits via telephone-, video-, and internet-based models on quality of life among adult asthma patients (McLean et al. 2011). The meta-analysis disclosed clinically significantly improved quality of life and reduced hospital readmission risk, particularly among participants with severe asthma symptoms.

In contrast, a systematic meta-analysis of 11 studies, including 1,460 patients in the intervention groups (mean age, 34.4 to 54.6 years) and 1,349 in the control groups (mean age, 30.7 to 56.4 years), with a treatment duration of 0.5 to 12 months (Zhao et al., 2015). The meta-analysis of the six eligible studies revealed no significant difference in asthma symptom score change between the telemedicine and control groups (g = 0.34; 95% confidence interval [CI], −0.05 to 0.74; Z = 1.69; p = 0.090). Although telemedicine interventions did not improve asthma function scores above those of controls in these studies, the authors considered other potential benefits of telemedicine to include long-term control of symptom exacerbation and decreased frequency of hospital admissions (Zhao et al., 2015).

There is a consensus that telemedicine offers considerable advantages to people who live in rural areas (e.g., Branning & Vater, 2016; CDC, 2020; Chongmelaxme et al., 2019; McLean et al. 2011). For example, Brown et al. (2017) conducted a prospective cohort pilot study to evaluate patients' satisfaction with telehealth delivery for asthma education in a rural, medically underserved North Dakota community. Analysis of the survey responses supported the notion that asthma education delivered via telemedicine technology was well received by the study participants. Although older participants took longer to adapt to using the technology than those who were younger, overall, most asthmatics in this rural community found telehealth technology a convenient way to access a specialty provider for disease education.

Along the same lines, two other studies examined the efficacy of telemedicine in allergic asthma symptom control among residents in remote rural communities (Cyr et al., 2019; Taylor et al., 2019). The findings of one study demonstrated that rural patients could receive telemedicine visits either in ambulatory and emergency department settings or using in-patient consults when allergy specialists are not readily available (Taylor et al., 2019). In the other study, telemedicine interventions yielded asthma outcomes that were comparable to those of but less costly than in-person visits and eliminated the inconvenience of travel from rural communities to urban centers (Cyr et al., 2019). These findings further support the conclusion that telemedicine is a cost-containing, effective solution to the shortage of specialty care in rural communities.

Chapter Summary

One in 13 people in the United States has asthma, making this disease one of the most prevalent conditions in the country (CDC,

2017). Asthma presents considerable health and economic burdens to patients, their families, and society (CDC, 2017; Nunes et al., 2017), making effective disease treatment and management a healthcare priority. However, barriers to care, such as a lack of transportation, lack of primary care physicians, and limited resources, often make it difficult for asthmatic patients to receive conventional face-to-face health care.

Overall, published evidence supports telemedicine's inclusion as a treatment method in managing adult asthmatic patients in inner-city and rural communities. Telemedicine can positively affect healthcare delivery across time and distance by expanding access, facilitating information exchange, and delivering care in alternate formats (Alvandi, 2017; Leath et al., 2018). However, multiple barriers to adopting telemedicine remain in rural and underserved inner-city communities, such as unfamiliarity with technology, poor mobile networks, and privacy concerns (Almathami et al., 2020; Duclos et al., 2017). Nonetheless, multiple researchers (e.g., Brown et al., 2017; Cyr et al., 2019; Taylor et al., 2019) have argued in favor of telemedicine, citing dramatic reduction in healthcare costs, increased access to specialty services, increased patient satisfaction, and improved health outcomes in rural and metropolitan areas of the United States and worldwide. The main benefits of telemedicine for patients with asthma are related to its potential to improve health outcomes and reduce associated economic burden on patients, their families, and society.

3

METHODOLOGY

Asthma is a chronic condition that disproportionately affects adults in inner-city, underserved populations (John et al., 2017). People from these communities often have difficulty accessing health care because of a lack of transportation or other barriers. Therefore, telemedicine represents an important alternative source of health care for people in underserved communities (Jong et al., 2019). This project specifically explored how telemedicine affects inner-city adults who have asthma. Through a systematic review of the published literature regarding the influence of telemedicine on long-term health outcomes, the project addressed three primary research questions:

1. In underserved adults (18 to 55 years old) with asthma, what is the effect of telemedicine conferences compared with face-to-face office visits on self-reported quality of life?
2. Compared with face-to-face treatment, how effective is telemedicine in decreasing asthma morbidity among underserved inner- city adults (18 to 55 years old)?
3. Compared with face-to-face specialist treatment, how effective is telemedicine in decreasing asthma mortality among underserved inner- city adults (18 to 55 years old)?

This chapter (Chapter 3) presents the study design, the target population, data collection methods, data analysis procedures, and limitations of the research design.

Study Design

The purpose of this project was to conduct a systematic review of the literature regarding the effects of telemedicine on inner-city adults with asthma. Systematic literature reviews allow researchers to search and analyze the existing literature on a particular subject (Chandler et al., 2021). For review, I selected articles that fit the pre-determined eligibility criterion (Appendix A) and then performed a quality assessment on each article to determine its inclusion (or not) in the review (Chandler et al., 2021). Systematic reviews are conducted according to a strict preestablished protocol, thereby minimizing researcher-induced bias. Because my goal was to comprehensively review of the available literature regarding the effects of telemedicine on underserved asthmatic populations, a systematic literature review is an appropriate choice of methodology.

In contrast, other methodologic approaches were deemed to be inappropriate for this project. For example, quantitative methods are used to explore the relationship between two variables (Punch, 2013). Given that the questions for this project involved a single phenomenon only (i.e., the use of telemedicine to treat asthma in inner-city adults), quantitative methods are an unsuitable approach. In addition, I discounted qualitative approaches such as phenomenological and case-study designs because my project goal was to comprehensively review the existing literature rather than to generate new data (Rubin & Rubin, 2012).

Types of Studies for Inclusion and Exclusion

This systematic literature review included quantitative and qualitative studies of the effects of telemedicine on inner-city adult populations with asthma. Randomized controlled trials, interventional trials, and non-randomized trials were included, as were studies that were case studies or observational. Additional inclusion criteria were publication in English between January 1, 2013, and May 31, 2021; a target population that comprised adults who had been diagnosed with asthma and lived in an inner-city setting; and evaluation of the effects of telemedicine on this target population. Studies in languages other than English, that focused on asthmatic adults who lived elsewhere than in an inner-city area, or that did not assess the effects of telemedicine on the desired target population were excluded. All relevant studies had at least one telemedicine outcome endpoint, such as an effect on a long-term health outcome, mortality, or morbidity. The definition of telemedicine used by the Cochrane review of telemedicine interventions for asthma was used as the basis for inclusion (McLean et al., 2011). In addition, only empirical studies that were published in peer-reviewed journals were included in the review; studies that were solely theoretical in nature or part of a dissertation, report, or other publication type were excluded.

Data Collection

Because this project was a systematic review of existing literature and did not involve study on human subjects, Institutional Review Board approval was unnecessary. The PubMed, Google Scholar, Web of Science, Medline, ClinicalTrials.gov, and Cumulative Index to Nursing and Allied Health Literature (CINAHL) databases were searched for relevant articles published during the time frame of January 1, 2013, through May 31, 2021. Strings of keywords and phrases (Table 1) in various combinations were used to search each of the databases to identify articles for potential review.

Table 1

Databases, Keywords, and Phrases Used to Identify Articles for Review

Database	Keywords or phrases
CINAHL	Telemedicine impact on asthma treatment
ClinicalTrials.gov	Telemedicine and asthma patient satisfaction
Google Scholar	Asthma and long-term telemedicine outcome
Medline	Telemedicine and asthma underserved population
PubMed	Telemedicine and asthma treatment "inner-city"
Web of Science	Telemedicine asthma self-management

Note: Each keyword phrase in the table was used to search each of the listed databases.

The study selection process (Figure 8) was done in alignment with the Preferred Reporting Items for Systematic Reviews and Meta-analyses (PRISMA) guidelines.

Figure 8

Process and Flow of the Systematic Literature Review in the Current Project

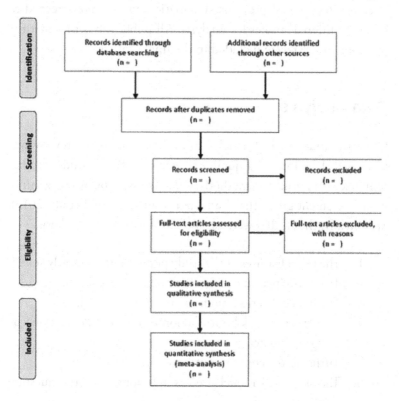

Note: The protocol used was adapted from the PRISMA flow diagram (Moher et al., 2009).

The number of records identified during the initial electronic search of each database was recorded in Excel. After all databases were searched, duplicate publications were excluded. Remaining studies were then screened for inclusion or exclusion based on the article title. The next step in the process was to screen articles by using their abstracts; when an article's inclusion or exclusion eligibility could not be determined according to the abstract, its full text was reviewed. In addition, the reference sections of all articles included in the review were screened manually, to maximize the number of relevant studies in the evaluation. Furthermore, the reference sections of previous systematic reviews were screened to solicit additional studies for analysis. All publications that met the inclusion criteria were included in the final synthesis.

Data Analysis

Once the final pool of articles to be included in the review was identified, I performed a quality assessment of each study. Studies that used quantitative methods were assessed by using a nine-item assessment guide that I adapted from Lagerveld et al. (2010). Specifically, the studies were assessed for the following criteria:

1. The main features of the study population are clearly stated.
2. The participation or response rate is at least 50%.
3. The data collection methods are clearly described.
4. Criteria such as job satisfaction or burnout are assessed by using a validated instrument.
5. Turnover or retention outcomes are clearly defined.
6. The statistical model used is appropriate for the question being answered.
7. The statistical significance of associations is tested and reported.
8. The study controlled for relevant confounding variables.
9. The number of cases in the study was at least 10 times the number of independent variables.

One point was given for each criterion met, with a maximum of nine points awarded per article. Studies with one to four points were rated as being of fair quality, those scoring five to seven points were of good quality and obtaining seven or more points were rated as being excellent.

Studies that used qualitative methods were assessed by using the nine-question tool in Hawker et al. (2002). Specifically, studies were assessed against the following criteria:

1. Abstract and title: Do they provide a clear description of the study?
2. Introduction and aims: Is there a good description of the background and clear statement of the aims of the research?
3. Method and data: Are the methods appropriate and clearly explained?
4. Sampling: Is the sampling strategy appropriate to address the aims?
5. Data analysis: Is the description of the data analysis sufficiently rigorous?
6. Ethics and bias: Have ethical issues been addressed, and was necessary ethical approval gained? Has the relationship between researchers and participants been adequately considered?
7. Results: Is there a clear statement of the findings?
8. Transferability or generalizability: Are the findings of this study transferable (generalizable) to a wider population?
9. Implications and usefulness: How important are these findings to policy and practice?

Each of the nine questions in this tool were answered as 'good,' 'fair,' 'poor,' or 'very poor.' After the tool was applied to each study selected for full-text review, scores were given a numerical value from one (very poor) to four (good), so that each study received a minimum of nine points and a maximum of 36 points. Studies with a total score between 32 and 36 received an overall rating of 'good,' those with a total score of 26 to 31 received an overall rating of 'fair,' studies with a total score between 21 to 25 were ranked as 'poor,' and those with an overall score of 25 or less were 'very poor.'

To address issues relating to potential research biases, each article selected for inclusion was screened independently by a second rater. Each rater independently performed quality assessments of each article, after which the final quality assessment score was determined by consensus. After both raters had read the full text of the included articles, they inductively developed various themes and codes by consensus during several meetings.

The characteristics and results of the studies that underwent the quality assessment were compiled into a table. Entered data included the title, year of publication, and authors of the article; the journal in which it was published; the type and design of the study; and its location, objectives, sample population, sample size, results, and limitations (Table 2).

Table 2
Data Extraction Table

Study Title	Year Published	Authors	Journal	Type of Study/ Design	Location	Objective	Sample Population	Sample Size	Results	Limitations	Funded? (Yes or No)	Study Duration

Each study was summarized to highlight how the use of telemedicine influenced long-term health outcomes, asthma self-management, and patient satisfaction in the sample population. Depending on the quality of the data gathered and assessed during this review, conclusions, and recommendations regarding the use of telemedicine as a treatment intervention for inner-city adults with asthma were made.

Limitations

Systematic literature reviews are effective ways to gain familiarity with the evidence available regarding a particular outcome or phenomenon. The approach helped minimize researcher bias by adhering to strict protocols; it could also help to establish the generalizability and consistency of findings across populations and treatment groups (Garg et al., 2008). However, as with all research approaches, systematic reviews have limitations. The first is that systematic reviews and meta-analyses cannot overcome the problems and limitations that exist within the original studies that they include (Garg et al., 2008). In other words, the shortcomings that are inherent in the existing literature persist in the systematic review.

In addition, systematic reviews need to be conducted with sufficient rigor, but determining just how much rigor is enough can be difficult (Garg et al., 2008). Common methodologic flaws in systematic reviews are the failure to avoid bias in study inclusion and the failure to assess the methodologic quality of the original studies (Mrkobrada et al., 2008). To minimize the effects of these limitations, the present review was guided by the PRISMA method, a commonly used protocol for the development of systematic literature reviews (Moher et al., 2009). In addition, each study included in the final review underwent quality assessment by using tools that have been widely used in other reviews.

Delimitations

As previously explained, the scope of this systematic review was restricted to studies published during 2013 and later. The fields of telemedicine and asthma treatment are rapidly evolving, therefore including only the most recent studies helped to maximize the relevance of the conclusions drawn from the review. In addition, the project was delimited to studies that were published in English, peer-reviewed journals. Furthermore, only studies that examined the outcomes of telemedicine on asthmatic adults living in inner-city areas were included; studies that did not include telemedicine as an intervention or in which the sample population did not reside in inner-city areas were excluded.

Project Summary

The purpose of this project was to conduct a systematic review of the effects of telemedicine applications on the long-term health benefits, morbidity, and mortality rates of inner-city American adults diagnosed with asthma. The literature examined was published between January 1, 2013, through May 31, 2021. Because asthma is one of the most prevalent chronic diseases in the United States and a major source of economic burden to patients, companies, and governments, the results of this study likely will have important ramifications on American society at large. Because telemedicine can be an effective alternative for people who lack means of transportation or who otherwise would have difficulty obtaining in-person medical care, whether incorporating telemedicine into the care of adult asthmatics residing in underserved inner-city communities reduces the symptoms and severity of asthma needs to be understood.

A systematic review of the literature addressing the use of telemedicine to treat asthmatic adults from inner-city populations was conducted. The review followed PRISMA guidelines and focused on studies published in English-language, peer-reviewed journals between January 1, 2013, and May 30, 2021, that specifically measured the effectiveness of telemedicine interventions on inner-city asthmatic adults. Articles were sourced from the Google Scholar, PubMed, Web of Science, ClinicalTrials.gov, Medline, and CINAHL databases and underwent quality assessment before their inclusion in the final analysis. The results of this study may enhance awareness of the benefits of telemedicine and provide practitioners a comprehensive review of the data regarding telemedicine's effectiveness in treating asthma.

RESULTS

Results

The systematic review of English-language literature followed the PRISMA guidelines to identify studies reporting outcomes associated with including telemedicine in the care of underserved adults (18 to 55 years old) with mild to severe chronic asthma. The initial search of the six selected databases returned 1,012 articles published between January 1, 2013, through May 31, 2021, and yielded 608 citations after duplicates were removed. This number was reduced to 57 after inclusion and exclusion criteria were applied by screening the article's title and abstract with specific keywords (Figure 9). Of these 57 articles, 46 were excluded after full-text screening. From the 11 articles remaining at this point, six were excluded during data extraction, leaving five peer-reviewed, full-text publications for analysis and synthesis within this systematic review (Figure 9).

Figure 9

Selection and Exclusion of Articles for the Systematic Literature Review

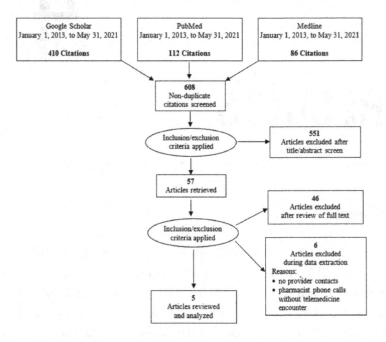

Note: Diagram of article selection during the systematic literature review, with reasons for exclusion.

Double coding was utilized for the 11 studies that passed full-text screening, and inter-rater agreement regarding the inclusion or exclusion of each of these studies in the systematic literature review was assessed through kappa analysis. The kappa statistic (κ) is the statistical tool typically used to determine agreement beyond chance between two or more observers when the observation of interest is categorical (Dettori & Norvell, 2020). The agreement coefficient, the κ value, can range from 0.81 to 1.0 (nearly perfect agreement) to ≤ 0.2 (equivalent to chance) (Dettori & Norvell, 2020). The higher the κ value, the stronger the agreement between raters and increased validity of the results; low κ values indicate poor inter-rater agreement. In particular, the inter-rater reliability for each of the five studies ultimately included for analysis was 'near perfect,' at a κ of 1.0 (Appendix B). Precise alignment was obtained between the two raters on all screening questions (Appendix C) for each of the five studies included for review (Table 3).

Table 3

Kappa Analysis for the Five Studies Included for Review

	Inclusion criteria present & exclusion criteria absent in study	Inclusion criteria absent & exclusion criteria absent in study	Subtotal
Inclusion criteria present & exclusion criteria absent in study	7	0	7
Inclusion criteria absent & exclusion criteria present in study	0	0	0
Subtotal	7	0	7

Note: The κ calculation is not shown for each of the 5 studies because all values and sums were the same for all studies. Inter-rater reliability had a κ value of 1 for all five of the included studies.

Both raters agreed to exclude the remaining six of the 11 studies from the review (Table 4). Precise alignment was not achieved for any of the six excluded studies (Appendix D).

49

Table 4

Kappa Analysis for the Six Excluded Studies

	Inclusion criteria present & exclusion criteria absent in study	Inclusion criteria absent & exclusion criteria present in study	Subtotal
Inclusion criteria present & exclusion criteria absent in study	5	2	7
Inclusion criteria absent & exclusion criteria present in study	4	3	7
Subtotal	9	5	14

Note: The inter-rater reliability for six excluded studies was associated with a κ value of 0.14.

The five studies that met the inclusion and exclusion criteria included a total of 607 participants, comprising adults (age, 18 to 55 years) with mild to severe asthma who received telemedicine intervention for symptom management with reported outcomes regarding asthma symptom control, such as confirmed cases of decreased asthma symptom flares, decreased hospitalization, decreased use of nebulizers, increased exercise tolerance, and improved quality of life. Two studies were randomized control trials, two were prospective cohort studies, and one was a contextual ground interventional study. Articles that reported pharmacist contact through phone calls without telemedicine encounters by healthcare providers or that described participants who were in rural regions without reported telemedicine end outcomes were excluded from the review. All five studies focused on telemedicine outcomes and effectiveness in the care of adults with mild to severe asthma in real-world settings, demonstrating telemedicine's influence in significantly improving participants' overall quality of life.

Of the five studies, one was published in 2013, one in 2015, one in 2018, one in 2019, and another in 2020. In addition, three studies were performed in the United States, one in Turkey, and the remaining one in the Netherlands. The United States is a crucial proponent in advancing telemedicine as an alternative healthcare source for people who might have difficulty accessing traditional forms of health care because of transportation-associated or other issues. Three of the five reviewed studies were completed in the United States, indicating that the United States accounts for the majority of research regarding telemedicine effectiveness in uncontrolled asthma outcomes among populations with difficulties receiving routine health care.

Gaalen et al. (2013) published a randomized controlled trial study, with data from Leiden and the Hague (2011–2013), conducted in the Netherlands. The study compared an 'internet group' of participants with those receiving usual care (face-to-face). A focus on the long-term outcomes were associated with internet-based comprehensive self-management strategies delivered to patients with uncontrolled asthma in primary care who required inhaled corticosteroids for more than three months during the previous year. The study occurred between November 2007 and July 2010 and included 101 adults (18 to 50 years old) in the internet group and 99 in the usual care (face-to-face) control group. Participants in the internet group received internet-based self-management (IBSM) support, including encounters with providers, which included group education sessions that focused on topics related to asthma self-management, use of the IBSM tool, and creation of an action plan involving current medication. In contrast, participants in the control group received standard asthma management intervention from health providers according to the Dutch College of General Practitioner, including a written action plan and a medical review at least once a year. After 12 months of baseline encounters, participants in the internet group showed significant improvement of health outcomes, demonstrated by increased Asthma-related Quality of Life (AQL) score (0.37; 95% CI, 0.14 to 0.61) and asthma control (−0.57; 95% CI, 00.88 to 0.26) as compared with UC face-to-face asthma standard management intervention. Within the same study, participants who remained for 30 months and received the internet-based intervention experienced an increase in their AQL score (0.34; 95% CI, 0.06 to 0.61) in favor of the IG group detected. In addition, the AQL score between 0 and 12 months of internet-group participants (0.43) did not differ significantly from the 30-month score of nonparticipants who received usual care (0.33).

Cingi et al. (2015) published a prospective randomized controlled double-blinded trial study. The goal was to investigate the effects of a mobile patient online engagement application on health outcomes and quality of life in patients with allergic rhinitis or asthma patients. This multicenter prospective study was conducted from June through December 2013, with data collection in Turkey. A total of 327 patients diagnosed with persistent allergic rhinitis or mild-to-severe persistent asthma were randomized into two intervention groups and two control groups upon their admission at outpatient clinics. The intervention groups received a mobile phone application (Physician On-call Patient Engagement Trial [POPET]), enabling them to communicate with their physician and record their health status and medication compliance. Participants with allergic rhinitis completed the Rhinitis Quality of Life Questionnaire (RQLQ) at admission and during the first month of the study. Participants with asthma groups completed the Asthma Control Test (ACT) at admission and during the third month of the study.

Among participants with allergic rhinitis, the online-encounter group showed better clinical improvement than the control group in terms of the overall quality of life score and measures of general problems, activity, and symptom control ($p < 0.05$). In addition, more asthmatic patients in the online-encounter group (49%) achieved a well-controlled asthma score (ACT >19) compared with the control group (27%), indicating a statistically significant ($p <$ 0.05) improvement in overall asthma symptom control.

Rasulnia et al. (2018) performed a prospective cohort study to examine the effectiveness of a remote digital coaching program on asthma control and patient experience. Study data were collected from May 2017 through July 2017. Included participants were 18 to 50 years old with current uncontrolled asthma, indicated by albuterol use more than twice weekly or requiring systematic corticosteroids. Fifty-one adults with uncontrolled asthma participated in a 12-week patient-centered remote digital platform. The coaching program used a combination of educational pamphlets, symptom trackers, best peak flow establishment, physical activity, and dietary counseling, in addition, the program coaches vigorously motivated disease self-management through telephone calls, texts, and emails. Baseline and post-intervention measures were quality of life, spirometry, ACT score, Asthma Symptom Utility Index score, rescue albuterol use, and exacerbation history.

Among the 51 patients recruited to receive the online-based coaching, 40 completed the study; eight subjects required assistance reading medical materials. Significant improvements from baseline were observed for patient-reported outcomes of Measurement Information System mental status ($p = 0.010$), body weight, and outpatient exacerbation frequency ($p = 0.028$). The changes from baseline in the ACT ($p = 0.005$) were statistically significant but did not achieve the pre-specified minimum clinically important difference; however, the change in the Asthma Symptom Utility Index score met both criteria. Spirometry and rescue albuterol use did not differ between baseline and study end.

Mammen et al. (2019) published a contextual grounded interventional study, for which the rationale was to determine whether clinical integration of smartphone telemedicine interventions into the care of adults with asthma improved symptom control, quality of life, and patient satisfaction rate. The participants in the study included seven adults (age, 18 to 40 years) with uncontrolled asthma who spoke English and owned a smartphone. The participants were patients who received care at an urban safety-net resident-run primary care clinic in western New York. Data collection for the study occurred between March and June 2019.

The intervention incorporated symptom monitoring by smartphone, smartphone telemedicine visits and self-management training with a nurse, and clinical decision-support software, which provided automated calculations of asthma severity, control, and stepwise therapy. The participants engaged in a 3-month beta-test. Asthma outcomes (control, quality of life, forced expiratory volume [FEV1]) and healthcare utilization patterns were measured at baseline and study end. Participants averaged four telemedicine visits each, resulting in a 94% patient satisfaction. All participants, who had uncontrolled asthma at the beginning of the study, achieved an end-of-study score of 5 (maximum, 7; classified as well-controlled). The mean asthma control score improved 1.55 points (0.59 to 2.51), quality of life improved 1.91 points (0.50 to 3.31), and FEV1 percent predicted increased 14.86% (3.09 to 32.80): effect sizes were 1.16, 1.09, and 0.96, respectively. In addition, preventive healthcare utilization increased significantly (1.86 visits annually compared with 0.28 for the prior year; 0.67 to 2.47), as did prescriptions for controller medications (9.29 prescriptions annually compared with 1.57 prescriptions annually previously; 4.85 to 10.58).

Mammen et al. (2020) completed a three-month mixed methods randomized trial study that incorporated a trained research assistant for data collection between 2018 and 2020. The study's objective was to evaluate the efficacy, feasibility, and acceptability of a multi-component smartphone telemedicine program to deliver asthma care remotely, support provider adherence to asthma management guidelines, and improve patient outcomes. Participants were adults (age 18 to 44 years) with a diagnosis of uncontrolled asthma who were recruited from a safety-net practice in upstate New York. At baseline, 80% of participants had uncontrolled asthma, but by 6 months, 80% were classified as well-controlled. Measure of asthma control and quality of life showed large increases (d = 1.955 and d = 1.579, respectively). FEV1 percentage predicted increased 4.2% (d = 1.687), with the greatest gain among men, smokers, and participants with a lower educational status. Provider adherence to national guidelines increased from 43.3% to 86.7% (95% CI, 22.11 to 64.55) and patient adherence to medication increased from 45.58% to 85.29% (95% CI, 14.79 to 64.62). Acceptability was 95.7%; in follow-up interviews, 29 of the 30 patients and 6 providers indicated the smartphone telemedicine intervention worked better than usual face-to-face care, supported effective self-management, and reduced symptoms over time, thus leading to increased self-efficacy and motivation to manage asthma. No other significant differences in intervention effects based on gender, smoking status, education, race/ethnicity, or presence of comorbid mental illness emerged. Improvement in quality of life was strongly associated with improved control (r = 0.80, p < 0.001) but not with FEV1 percentage predicted (r = 0.087, p = 0.648). Similarly, the results of t-testing indicated that the Asthma Control Questionnaire score decreased significantly over time, whereas both the Asthma Quality of Life score and FEV1 percentage predicted increased over time, indicating improved asthma control, quality of life, and pulmonary function.

Analyzing the similarities of the five articles synthesized in the systematic review revealed key recurring themes. Telemedicine application in the care of adult participants with asthma who lived in metropolitan or urban areas yielded reports of reduced asthma symptoms, increased medications adherence, successful tobacco cessation, increased satisfaction with asthma care, decreased frequency of emergency room visits and hospitalizations, and improved quality of life. The findings support the increased incorporation of telemedicine into the care of underserved inner-city adults with asthma. For these patients, telemedicine offers significant long-term health benefits within the United State and worldwide.

In-depth data from the five reviewed studies are included in Appendix E.

Excluded Studies

The two reviewers excluded six articles after viewing their full texts. The most common reasons for exclusion were participant age, rural residents, and that the intervention did not meet the inclusion criteria. Often studies were excluded because the intervention did not include telemedicine end-outcomes measures or because participants had no face-to-face or telemedicine engagement with a primary care physician but only phone calls from pharmacists.

Effectiveness Measures Due to Telemedicine

Two of the five analyzed studies concluded effectiveness of telemedicine. In the study by Rasulnia et al. (2018), the specific effectiveness of telemedicine in the care of adults (age, 18 to 55 years) with uncontrolled asthma emerged as a decrease in acute worsening asthma symptoms, improved asthma medication compliance, successful tobacco cessation, and a clinically significant decrease in the ACT score ($p = 0.005$). To add to the conclusions of the Rasulnia et al. (2018) study, & Cingi et al. (2015) also cited telemedicine effectiveness as a significant improvement in patient satisfaction with asthma symptom control, which correlated with more telemedicine patients (49%) achieving a well-controlled asthma score (ACT > 19) compared with the control group (27%; $P < 0.05$). Both studies reported the effectiveness of telemedicine on asthma management.

Outcome Measures Due to Telemedicine

Three studies included in the review focused on adult outcomes associated with telemedicine, namely reduced asthma symptoms, improved quality of life, and improved morbidity and mortality (Gaalen et al., 2013; Mammen et al. 2019; Mammen et al. 2020).

For example, compared with their peers who received standard, face-to-face care, participants in the internet-based treatment group showed increased Asthma-related Quality of Life scores at 0.37 (95% CI, 0.14 to 0.61) and asthma control at −0.57 (95% CL 00.88 to 0.26) as compared with the standard face-to-face asthma management intervention.

In addition, the mean asthma control score improved 1.55 points (CI ¼, 0.59 to 2.51), the asthma quality of life score improved 1.91 points (CI ¼, 0.50 to 3.31), and FEV1 percentage predicted increased 14.86% (CI ¼, 3.09 to 32.80); effect sizes were 1.16, 1.09, and 0.96, respectively (add your sources). Furthermore, preventive healthcare utilization increased significantly to 1.86 visits per year compared with 0.28 per year previously with 95% CI, 0.67 to 2.47, as did prescriptions for controller medications with 9.29 prescriptions per year compared with 1.57 prescriptions per year previously based on 95% CI, 4.85 to 10.58 (Gaalen et al. 2013; Mammen et al. 2019; Mammen et al. 2020). The data from these studies show the benefit of telemedicine on increasing adherence to asthma treatment and preventive services.

Study Findings Related to Research Questions

Undertreatment of asthma, limited access to care, and overall poor asthma outcomes prevail across the United States and globally. People with uncontrolled asthma are at increased risk of morbidity and mortality, diminished quality of life, and elevated symptom burden (Mammen et al., 2020). Ways to improve clinical care and asthma outcomes for underserved residents are needed. Patients and physicians have started to use online communications, and the potential of mobile or internet-based applications to support health care for underserved adults with uncontrolled asthma is rapidly becoming realized (Cingi et al., 2015). Internet-based technology is an appealing medium for asthma management, especially for underserved populations. For example, providing an IBSM support program to patients with moderate or severe uncontrolled persistent asthma for one-year improved asthma-related quality of life, asthma control, lung function, and the number of symptom-free days, compared with usual care or face-to-face intervention visits (Mammen et al., 2020). However, this review chose to evaluate the effectiveness of telemedicine in the care of underserved asthmatic adults (18 to 55 years old), which provided literature support to the objectives and the three research questions in this project.

Regarding research question 1—In underserved inner-city adults (18 to 55 years old) with asthma, what is the effect of telemedicine conferences compared with face-to-face office visits on self-reported quality of life? —3 of the 5 studies included in the systematic review reported pertinent data. Findings from these studies demonstrated significantly improved outcomes in favor of the telemedicine group in various ways. For example, telemedicine participants had better asthma-related quality of life and asthma symptom control at one year than those who received standard care. In addition, participants who were followed at 30 months showed further significant improvements in both asthma-related quality of life and asthma control scores. No such differences were demonstrated for the control group, who were treated with inhaled corticosteroids and whose lung function was measured according to FEV1 (Mammen et al., 2020).

Participants in the internet group reported enhancement in knowledge regarding asthma symptom management and developed strategies for self-monitoring and asthma action plans. Regular medication reviews ensured the accuracy of dosages, decreased the numbers of hospitalizations, and limited unplanned emergency room visits in 30 months after baseline study. Furthermore, telemedicine participants reported improved knowledge about the disease process of asthma, saying that it enhanced communication with their healthcare provider, increased medication adherence, and enhanced engagement in asthma care (Mammen et al., 2020).

Regarding other measures of telemedicine effectiveness, participants' ability to use and willingness to accept the technology increased over time (mean score = 6.61; 1 SD = 0.47). Many participants reported that the telemedicine intervention "changed their life," enabling them to take control of their asthma and became more active, and that they felt "like a regular person for the first time in their adult life" (Mammen et al., 2015).

In the study by Mazi et al. (2018), subjects participating in a telemedicine program reported significant improvements in asthma outcomes through diet and exercise that decreased the mean body mass index from baseline (34.9 kg/m^2) to post-study (33.8 kg/m^2; P = 0.056). Among 35 subjects reporting adherence to the intervention, 11 (31.4%) indicated that the program improved their asthma medication compliance. In addition, during the study, one (16.7%) of the five current smokers successfully quit using tobacco, and 21 subjects reported they had established their best peak expiratory flow rate.

Patients who received intervention through the POPET application showed significant overall improved clinical outcomes when compared with the controls (Cing et al., 2015). These measured outcome improvements were particularly noteworthy in areas where the questionnaires assessed patients' productivity, perception of disease, and emotions toward their disease state., More patients in the POPET-Asthma group (49%) achieved a well-controlled asthma score (ACT > 19) than in the control group (27%; p < 0.05). Furthermore, the total ACT score at the third month were significantly better for the POPET-Asthma patients compared with the control group (*p* < 0.05); the median improvement in the total ACT score was 6.0 points for the POPET-Asthma group and 2.0 points for the control group. Finally, patients in the POPET-Asthma group felt less impaired in their activities, used less rescue inhaler medication, and thought they had better control of their asthma (Cing et al., 2015). The findings from the studies discussed herein demonstrated the positive effects of telemedicine in terms of self-reported quality of life among adult patients with asthma compared with participants who had face-to-face office visits and did not experience decrease in asthma symptoms.

Regarding research question 2—Compared with face-to-face treatment, how effective is telemedicine in decreasing asthma morbidity among underserved inner- city adults (18 to 55 years old)? —80% of the participants had uncontrolled asthma at baseline of the study by Mammen et al. (2020). However, findings demonstrated an 80% improvement in asthma-related symptoms, including participant-reported decreased shortness of breath, wheezing, coughing, nighttime waking due to difficulty breathing. In addition, 29 of the 30 of participants said that the Technology Enabled Asthma Management program worked better to control acute exacerbation of their asthma-related symptoms than did their usual care. Thus, the study conclusions supported the effects of telemedicine on self-management and reduced uncontrolled symptoms over time and leading to greater self-efficacy and motivation for appropriate asthma self-management (Mammen et al., 2020). Individuals with uncontrolled asthma cases are at increased risk of morbidity, diminished quality of life, and worsened asthma burden; the findings described demonstrate telemedicine's potential to minimize these risks and decrease asthma morbidity among underserved inner-city adults (18 to 55 years old) compared with their peers who receive face-to-face visits.

Using the POPET application, 88% of participants completed the research trial and had significantly fewer unplanned hospital and emergency room visits ($p = 0.015$, $z = -2.438$), compared with the face-to-face group (Cing et al., 2015). In addition, as mentioned previously, more patients in the POPET-Asthma group (49%) achieved a well-controlled asthma score (ACT > 19) compared with the control group (27%). Furthermore, the total ACT score in the study's third month was significantly better for the POPET-Asthma patients ($p < 0.05$; Cing et al., (2015). Moreover, patients in the

POPET-Asthma group felt less impaired in their activities, used less rescue inhaler medication, and thought they had better control of their asthma, and more of those in the POPET-Asthma group completed the study than did those in the control, usual care group. Therefore, asthma morbidity was significantly decreased ($p < 0.05$) among telemedicine participants compared with those who received standard, face-to-face care from their healthcare providers. These findings indicated that telemedicine implementation in the care of underserved asthmatic adults (18 to 55 years) could significantly ameliorate asthma morbidity overall in the United States and other parts of the world.

For research question 3—Compared with face-to-face specialist treatment, how effective is telemedicine in decreasing asthma mortality among underserved inner- city adults (18 to 55 years old)? —all five studies included in the systematic review provided valuable data in this regard.

Mammen et al. (2020) cited limited access to care, improper treatment of asthma, and non-adherence to treatment recommendations as contributing factors. The prevalence of uncontrolled asthma cases is strongly associated with poor asthma outcomes across the United States and other parts of the world, thereby exposing persons with prevalent asthma symptoms to increased risk of diminished quality of life and mortality. In essence, telemedicine implementation in the care of underserved populations was concluded to improve asthma-related quality of life, asthma control, lung function, and increased the number of asthma-related by 80% (Mammen et al., 2020); increased the number of symptom-free days (Gaalen et al., 2013); ameliorated shortness of breath, wheezing, and coughing without difficulty breathing (Mazi et al., 2015; Mammen et al., 2018); enhanced knowledge regarding asthma symptom management, promoted the development of self-monitoring strategies and asthma action plans (Cingi et al., 2015); and reduced the numbers of unplanned hospitalization and emergency room visits (Cing et al., 2015; Mammen et al., 2018).

Together, these findings demonstrate that compared with face-to-face visits with a primary care physician or specialist, adding telemedicine to the care of underserved adults in the United States and worldwide has strong potential to decrease the risk of asthma-related mortality. By extension, the overall findings regarding the application of telemedicine to asthma care support the long-term benefits of this systematic review for underserved and general populations who are burdened with mild to severe asthma in the United States and globally.

Biases and Limitations of Included Studies

The published review outlined biases and limitations throughout the five studies included in the final analysis. Regarding potential biases, three of the included studies received financial support from research institutes and academic organizations. Gaalen et al. (2013) received grants from The Netherlands Organization for Health, Research, and Development (Zon-MW) and the Lung Foundation of the Netherlands; the authors also received funding for publication from the Netherland Organization Scientific Research (NOW) from an incentive fund for unrestricted-access publication. In addition, Mazi et al. (2018) obtained funding through a grant from Genentech, LLC, and Mammen et al. (2019) received financial support from Sigma Theta Tau nursing society, Epsilon Xi chapter. Additional reported biases and limitations include:

- Low response rate
- Non statistically significant difference in improved asthma symptoms and quality of life between telemedicine and usual-care groups
- High attrition rate in control group
- Short study period
- Small sample size

- ≥20% dropout rate
- Lack of cost analysis
- Study sample predominantly female
- Small sample size
- Participants younger, minority, lower socioeconomic status, lower health literacy
- Interventions by single provider
- Research-related incentive
- High frequency of follow-up visits

Summary of Systematic Literature Review Findings

This systematic literature review focused on the evidence supporting the use of telemedicine in management of asthma in inner-city adults aged 18 to 55 years. All five of the studies included in the systematic review reported the effectiveness of telemedicine on asthma symptom control, quality of life, improvement of FEV1, emergency room visits, and incidents of hospitalizations at baseline and end of the study. Results of the studies focused on the contributions of telemedicine in improving asthma quality of life and decreasing disease-associated morbidity and mortality. Two of the five studies assessed the effectiveness of telemedicine on asthma care for an underserved population based on prospective cohort or randomized control studies. Noted outcomes were related to a significant decrease in acute worsening asthma symptoms, improved asthma medication compliance, and successful tobacco cessation (Rasulnia et al., 2018). However, in one study (Rasulnia et al., 2018), baseline peak flow at end of study did not differ between telemedicine participants and the control group. In addition, results of another study (Cingi et al., 2015) noted a statistically significant improvement in patient satisfaction, with more telemedicine patients obtaining improved control of asthma-related symptoms (49% compared with 27% of the control group; $p < 0.05$) and achieving a well-controlled asthma score (ACT > 19; $P < 0.05$).

Together, findings from the systematic review demonstrated the substantial impact of telemedicine on health outcomes and quality of life in asthma, potentially through decreases in the number of hospital admissions and repeat physician visits and in losses in productivity. The systematic review synthesis included two randomized control trials. In the mixed method randomized trial conducted by Mammen et al. (2020), the researchers examined telemedicine effectiveness in delivering asthma care remotely via smartphone to underserved young adults (age 18 to 44) living with chronic uncontrolled asthma in urban upstate New York. The study demonstrated a profound reduction in asthma symptoms among study participants, with a considerably improved quality of life. At baseline, 80% of participants had uncontrolled asthma, but by 6 months into the trial, 80% of the participants' asthma showed significant clinical improvement, with symptoms reported to be well controlled. In addition, telemedicine recipients reported improvements in asthma control and quality of life (d = 1.955 and d = 1.579, respectively; Mammen et al., 2020).

In the second randomized controlled trial, the researchers investigated the effectiveness of a mobile telemedicine patient engagement application on health outcomes and quality of life in urban adults (age, 18 to 50 years) living with uncontrolled asthma in the Netherlands (Gaalen et al., 2013). The study's results showed significant improvement in asthma symptom control and asthma-related quality of life (Gaalen et al., 2013). In addition, Gaalen et al. concluded that telemedicine recipients who remained in the study at 30 months after baseline continued to show significant improvement in terms of asthma-related quality of life (0.29; 95% CI, 0.01 to 0.57) and asthma control (−0.33; 95% CI, −0.61 to −0.05). The synthesis of the results from both trials answers all three research questions and demonstrates telemedicine's potential to improve asthma quality of life and decrease disease-associated morbidity and mortality for current populations with chronic uncontrolled symptoms.

In summary, the implementation of telemedicine in the care of asthmatic adults (18 to 55 old) living with asthma in urban and metropolitan areas in the United States, the Netherlands, and Turkey demonstrated significant effectiveness in asthma symptom control, increased quality of life, reduced emergency room visits, and significantly decreased in hospitalization, measured as approximately 80% improvement in symptom control and 0.38% improvement in asthma-related quality of life at 6 to 30 months after baseline treatment initiation. The findings support telemedicine's potential contribution to enhancing the lives of underserved inner-city asthmatic adults (18 to 55 years old). Once telemedicine is incorporated into patients' care plans, it will help to improve quality of life and decrease asthma symptoms, morbidity, and mortality. Furthermore, this systematic review study validated telemedicine's long-term health benefits for underserved asthmatic patients in the United States and globally.

DISCUSSION

The data from this systematic review demonstrated that telemedicine intervention is a crucial and effective approach to supplement primary and specialist care. Telemedicine is concluded to improve access to healthcare for underserved populations with mild to uncontrolled asthma to improve disease outcomes in the United States and other parts of the world. The underlying importance of the telemedicine approach lies in its ability to reduce barriers to accessing primary or specialist asthma care. Telemedicine is inherently more flexible than in-office care. Bearing in mind that underserved populations have problems with transportations and mobility, a particular benefit of telemedicine applications is that patients are not required to travel to a particular location to participate in health care services. Therefore, extending telemedicine into patients' homes or communities via a readily available and familiar medium such as a smartphone, would essentially render more services for and become a frontliner for primary or specialist care delivery. Extended benefits would potentially lead to improving asthma symptom control, enhancing quality of life, and decreasing morbidity and mortality in patient suffering from asthma. Because of the ability to supersede geographic boundaries, telemedicine implementation in asthma care could increase the clinical reach to underserved asthma patients everywhere. In addition, telemedicine may become a key to delivering timely health care to populations with asthma in remote or underserved locations in the United States and throughout the world.

Several studies have demonstrated the use of remote monitoring, self-management training, telemedicine, smartphones, and computer decision-support software (CDSS) can improve health outcomes (Gaalen et al., 2013; Mammen et al.,2019). However, Mammen et al. (2019) was the first research group to combine abovementioned components into a single technological package that effectively integrates real-world medical practice and live electronic medical record systems into an integrated smartphone telemedicine program to deliver asthma care remotely. The large effect sizes of their crucial results (0.96 to 2.62), with marked improvement in outcomes, supported the integrated approach (Gaalen et al., 2013; Mammen et al., 2019). On average, telemedicine participants achieved a 15% increase in FEV1, crossing the critical clinical threshold of >80%. In addition, asthma control and quality of life associated with telemedicine use were 3 to 4 times higher than baseline (Mammen et al., 2019; Mammen et al., 2020).

To evaluate the long-term consequences of asthma patients' reminder systems and online intervention on medication adherence interventions and to understand the design implications of the engagement software, Cingi et al. (2015) developed the POPET application to assess the effect of a mobile patient engagement tool on clinical outcomes, especially the quality of life of asthma patients. At study baseline, all patients received recommended treatment guidelines and medications during office visits. However, the intervention groups also communicated with their physician by using the POPET system. About 92% of physicians responded to all urgent messages and serious health status submissions. With this intervention, due to increased physician access, satisfaction scores were significantly higher in the POPET group than for patients in the control group (Cingi et al., 2015). In addition, patients who used the POPET application required fewer office visits in comparison to the control group.

During the posttreatment period, the POPET group participants again had better results than the control group. In the POPET-Asthma group, more patients (49%) achieved a well-controlled asthma score (ACT > 19) compared with the control group (27%; Cingi et al., 2015). These findings support telemedicine intervention's significant contribution to improving asthma quality of life when skillfully integrated into the participant's intervention plan to enhance asthma outcomes.

Few studies have focused on the impact of digital intervention and telemedicine in asthma management for underserved populations (Cingi et al., 2015; Mammen et al., 2020; Rasulnia et al., 2018). However, the result of this review concluded the relevancy of digital coaching and telemedicine in asthma care for underserved populations, by offering them resources to enhance patient education, counseling to improve quality of life, and improved autonomy for self-care in asthma management. Through these measures, telemedicine minimizes the need for face-to-face encounters with clinicians for medication management and the number of required office visits.

Medication adherence is one of the most difficult challenges faced by patients burdened with poor asthma management. Rasulnia et al. (2018) and Cingi et al. (2015) considered that medication adherence was a crucial guideline that aided participants to determine the best peak flow and establish an asthma action plan, another management strategy that wass notoriously poor among asthma patients. In this context, more than half of the subjects were able to achieve their best peak flow rate—and for the first time (more than 50%). In addition, 25% of the research subjects reported that their medication adherence improved due to the medication adherence program. In summary, asthma medication adherence was crucial to enhancing asthma patients' quality of life and decreasing morbidity and mortality, the benchmarks for the current systematic review study.

This systematic review is unique given that it is one of the first to consider the effects of telemedicine implementation in the care of underserved adults (18 to 55 years old) with mild to chronic uncontrolled asthma and living in underserved regions in the United States and globally. Quality of life, morbidity, and mortality in the study population were followed as evaluable measures. The goal of the review was to obtain objective evidence regarding the benefits of telemedicine on asthma care among underserved adults and their health outcomes. Findings from this review cited published studies than had not been previously reviewed by using a systematic review method. The literature provided evidence that implementation of telemedicine in the care of underserved populations improved self-reported quality of life and decrease asthma-associated morbidity and mortality to a greater extent than what was initially anticipated.

Several limitations to this systematic review were due to the different study designs across the five included studies. For example, two studies were randomized controlled studies, which provided considerable insight into the research cause and effect relation with minimal bias and few confounding factors. However, the randomized control trial designed by Mammen et al. (2020) had limitations regarding the use of a small sample of low socioeconomic status, of urban young adult patients from a single hospital-based clinic, and of a single nurse practitioner to provide participant intervention. In addition, the study had a high frequency of participant follow-up visits, which materialized into increased participation and retention, resulting in a positive outcome bias.

Overall, analysis of the findings suggested that the broad generalizability and external validity of the study results may be limited, given the small sample size and demographics of the study population. Nevertheless, the data from the studies supported the benefits of telemedicine inclusion in the care of underserved adults with uncontrolled asthma, with the end goal of enhanced quality of life and decreased morbidity and mortality (Mammen et al., 2020).

The second randomized study (Gaalen et al., 2013) cited limitations of low response rate compared with other long-term outcome studies, which might limit the generalizability or external validity of our review results. This randomized trial indicates significant benefit of telemedicine in the treatment of underserved asthmatic adults, given that results at 12 months after baseline showed improved outcomes in favor of the telemedicine group as indicated by improvements asthma-related quality of life at (0.37; 95% CI, 0.14 to 0.61) and asthma control (–0.57; 95% CI, –0.88 to –0.26) as compared with the face-to-face care group (Gaalen et al., 2013). In addition, the responses of telemedicine participants revealed the relatively high quality of life and supported the conclusion that telemedicine implementation in the care of underserved asthmatic adults (18 to 55 years old) increased the quality of life and reduced disease-associated morbidity and mortality.

The prospective study by Cingi et al. (2015) noted the limitation of attrition rate in the control group. In addition, the number of subjects lost from the control group was higher than that number in the POPET group, despite the close communication between physician and patient. There was no discussed problem in following the patients. Rather, communication was more difficult in the control group, because of the lack of communication between the physicians and patients outside of office visits, thus leading to the higher attrition rate. Typically, patients prefer healthcare services that engage them and lead to open communication with timely feedback. Reflected in the POPET study, patients felt valued and supported through telemedicine physician–patient communications, making them willing to use the application and improving their overall quality of life outcomes. The study showed that using a mobile engagement platform, such as POPET, could considerably improve patients' health outcomes and quality of life, thus potentially decreasing the numbers of hospital admissions and repeated doctor' visits and loss in productivity. The most marked improvements in both disease groups (allergic rhinitis and asthma) were in domains related to activity, productivity, and perception of disease and emotion—all of which counted as outcomes of high importance to the patients.

In the other prospective study (Rasulnia et al., 2018), limitations such as short study duration, small sample size, 20% dropout rate, lack of cost analysis, and a study sample predominantly composed of women emerged as biases. A larger sample size and more extended intervention might have clearly demonstrated the benefit of acute care visits related to asthma. Women may be more likely than men to accept an intervention that promotes empowerment and self-management of asthma.

A particular strength of this systematic review was the stringency in the predefined study protocol, including its clearly defined inclusion and exclusion criteria, double coding, the protocol to minimize selection bias, and the numerous databases searched. The overall κ-value (1.0) for the studies included in the review demonstrated the strength of the double coding protocol. The significance of this value showed the extent to which the studies included in the review correctly represented the inclusion and exclusion criteria. Both raters extracted a few data points from within the paper and transcribed them into the data extraction tool to ensure a high degree of agreement with the outcome of the high κ-score.

CONCLUSIONS

Findings from this systematic review add to the body of knowledge regarding the effects of telemedicine in the care of inner-city, underserved adults (18 to 55 years old) with asthma. Previous research points to telemedicine as a beneficial alternative source of health care for underserved populations with asthma. Given the challenges due to transportation or mobility issues, these populations often described difficulty accessing traditional forms of health care. Consequently, telemedicine is likely to contribute to improving uncontrolled asthma outcomes; thereby, improving quality of life, and decreasing morbidity and mortality among such populations.

Few previous studies have specifically addressed the impact of telemedicine on improving quality of life, morbidity, and mortality in underserved, inner-city adults (18 to 55 years old) with asthma.

By addressing the research questions, the studies synthesized during this systematic review of the literature have hopefully narrowed the knowledge gap on the topic of interest. The evidence showed that underserved asthmatic patients whose care plans included telemedicine implementation had improved asthma-related quality of life, asthma control, and lung function in comparison to those patients who received traditional, face-to-face care. Currently, telemedicine services for adult asthma care in underserved populations of inner-city areas are sparse. The importance of including these services in health care plans, especially those of traditionally underserved populations, needs to be re-evaluated and further emphasized. In addition, community and health care leaders require effective strategies to enhance the asthma-related quality of life and decrease disease-associated morbidity and mortality among underserved adults with asthma in the United States and worldwide. Raising awareness of this issue is critical.

REFERENCES

Almathami, H. K. Y., Win, K. T., & Vlahu-Gjorgievska, E. (2019). Barriers and facilitators that influence telemedicine-based, real-time, online consultation at patients' homes: Systematic literature review. *Journal of Medical Internet Research*, *22*(2). https://doi.org/10.2196/16407

American Academy of Family Physicians. (2021). What is the difference between telemedicine and telehealth? https://www.aafp.org/news/media-center/kits/telemedicine-and-telehealth.html

American Lung Association. (2017). Asthma trends and burden. https://www.lung.org/research/ trends-in-lung-disease/ asthma-trends-brief/trends-and-burden

American Well. (2019). Telehealth index: 2019 consumer survey. https://static.americanwell.com/app/uploads/2019/07/American-Well-Telehealth-Index-2019-Consumer-Survey-eBook2.pdf

Alvandi, M., (2017). Telemedicine and its role in revolutionizing healthcare delivery. *American Journal of Accountable Care*, *5*(1). https://www.ajmc.com/view/telemedicine-and-its- role-in-revolutionizing-healthcare-delivery

Asher, I., Pearce, N., Strachan, D., Billo, N., Bissell, K., Chen-Yuan, C., Ellwood, P., Sony, E. A., García-Marcos, L., & Marks, G. (2018). The global asthma reports. Global Asthma Network. https://www.globalasthmareport.org

Bhaskar, S., Bradley, S., Chattu, V. K., Adisesh, A., Nurtazina, A., Kyrykbayeva, S., Sakhamuri, S., Yaya, S., Sunil, T., Pravin, T., Mucci, V., Moguilner, S., Israel-Korn, S., Alacapa, J., Mishra,

A., Pandya, S., Schroeder, S., Atreja, A., Banach, M., & Ray, D. (2020). Telemedicine across the globe—Position paper from the COVID-19 pandemic health system resilience program (REPROGRAM) [International Consortium]. *Frontiers in Public Health, 8.* https://doi.org/10.3389/fpubh.2020.556720

Bian, J., Cristaldi, K. K., Summer, A. P., Su, Z., Marsden, J., Mauldin, P.D., & McElligott, J. T. (2019). Association of a school-based, asthma-focused telehealth program with emergency department visits among children enrolled in South Carolina Medicaid. *JAMA Pediatrics, 173*(11), 1041–1048. 10.1001/jamapediatrics.2019.3073

Branning, G, & Vater, M, 2016). Healthcare spending: plenty of blame to go around. *American Health and Drug Benefit, 9*(8): 445–447. PMCID: PMC5394555

Breen, M. G., & Matusitz, J. (2010). An evolutionary examination of telemedicine: a health and computer-mediated communication perspective. *Social Work in Public Health 25*(1), 59– 71. https://doi.org/10.1080/19371910902911206

Brown, W., Schmitz, T., Scott, M. D., & Friesner, D. (2017). Is telehealth right for your practice and your patients with asthma? *Journal of Patient Practice, 4*(1), 46–49. https://doi.org/10.1177/2374373516685952

Centers for Disease Control and Prevention. (2020). Telehealth in rural communities. https://www.cdc.gov/chronicdisease/resources/publications/factsheets/telehealth-in-rural-communities.htm

Centers for Disease Control and Prevention (2017). National health interview survey (NHIS): National surveillance of asthma—United States. https://www.cdc.gov/asthma/nhis/default.htm

Centers for Disease Control and Prevention (CDC) (2018). CDC's most recent asthma data. https://www.cdc.gov/asthma/most_recent_data.htm

Center for Disease Control and Prevention (CDC) (2019). Asthma. .https://www.cdc.gov/asthma/default.htm.

Centers for Medicare and Medicaid Services (2020). Telemedicine seeks to improve a patient's health by permitting two-way, real time interactive communication between the patient and the physician or practitioner at the distant site. CMS.gov

Chandler, J., Cumpston, M., Thomas, J., Higgins, J. P. T., Deeks, J. J., Clarke, M. J. (2021) Chapter I: Introduction. In: Higgins J. P. T., Thomas J., Chandler J., Cumpston M., Li T., Page M. J., & Welch V. A. (Eds). Cochrane handbook for systematic reviews of interventions, version 6.2 (updated February 2021). Cochrane, 2021. www.training.cochrane.org/handbook

Chongmelaxme, B., Lee, S., Dhippayom, T., Saokaew, S., Chaiyakunapruk, N., Dilokthornsakul,

P. (2019). The effects of telemedicine on asthma control and patients' quality of life in adults: A systematic review and meta-analysis. *Journal of Allergy and Clinical Immunology*, 7(1), 199–216. https://doi.org/10.1016/j.jaip.2018.07.015

Cingi, Cperiod, Yorgancioglu, A., Cingi, C. C., Oguzulgen, K., Muluk, B. N., Ulusoy, K. S., Orhon, N., Yumru, C., Gokdag, D., Karakaya, G., Elebi, S. A., Obanoglu, H. B. C., Unlu, H., & Aksoy, M. A. (2015). The "physician on-call patient engagement trial" (POPET): Measuring the impact of a mobile patient engagement application on health outcomes and quality of life in allergic rhinitis and asthma patients. *International Forum of Allergy & Rhinology*. 5(6). 487-497. DOI: 10.1002/alr.21468

Cyr, M. E., Etchin, G. A., Guthrie, B. J., & Benneyan, J. C. (2019). Access to specialty healthcare in urban versus rural US populations: A systematic literature review. *BMC Health Services Research*, 19(974). https://doi.org/10.1186/s12913-019-4815-5

Dettori R.J, & Norvell D.C, (2020). Kappa and beyond: Is there agreement? *Global Spine Journal*, 10 (4). https://doi.org/10.1177/2192568220911648

Dinesen, B., Nonnecke, B., Lindeman, D., Toft, E., Kidholm, K., Jethwani, K., Young, H. M., Spindler, H., Oestergaard, U. C., Southard, A. J., Gutierrez, M., Anderson, N., & Nesbitt,

T. (2016). Personalized telehealth in the future: A global research agenda. *Journal of Medical Internet Research, 18*(3). https://doi. org/10.2196/jmir.5257

Dor, A., Luo, Q., Gerstein, M. T., Malveaux, F., Mitchell, H., & Markus, A. R. (2018). Cost- effectiveness of an evidence-based childhood asthma intervention in real-world primary care settings. *Journal of Ambulatory Care Management, 41*(3), 213–24.

Duos, V., Yé, M., Moubassira, K., Sanou, H., Sawadogo, N. H., Bibeau, G., & Sié, A. (2017) Situating mobile health: A qualitative study of mHealth expectations in the rural health district of Nouna, Burkina Faso. *Health Research Policy & Systems, 15*, 41-53. https://doi.org/10.1186/s12961-017-0211-y

Erquicia, S. P., Arenas, S. D., Landa, U. I., Basterrechea, A. I., Hernandez, Z., T, & Moreno, O.B. (2016). The impact of telemedicine in healthcare demand by patients with severe persistent asthma. *European Respiratory Journal, 48*. https://doi. org/10.1183/ 13993003.congress-2016.PA2892

Ferrer-Rocio, O., Garcia-Nogales, A., & Pelaez, C. (2010). The impact of telemedicine on quality of life in rural areas: the Extremadura model of specialized care delivery. *Telemedicine and e-Health, 16*(2), 233–43. https://doi.org/10.1089/tmj.2009.0107

Gaalen, J. L. V., Beerthuizen, T., Meer, V. D. V., Reisen, V. P., Geertje W. G., Snoeck-Stroband, J. S., & Sont, K. J. (2013). Long-term outcomes of internet-based self-management support in adults with asthma: randomized controlled trial. *Journal of Medical Internet Research, 15*(9): e188. doi: 10.2196/jmir.2640

Garg, A. X., Hackam, D., & Tonelli, M. (2008). Systematic review and meta-analysis: When one study is just not enough. *CJASN, 3*(1), 253-260. https://doi.org/10.2215/CJN.01430307.

Gergen, P. J., & Togias, A. (2015). Inner-city asthma. *Immunology and Allergy Clinics of North America, 35*(1), 101–114. https://doi. org/10.1016/j.iac.2014.09.006

George, S. M., Hamilton, A., & Baker, R. (2009). Pre-experience perceptions about telemedicine among African Americans and Latinos in South Central Los Angeles. *Telemedicine and e-Health, 15*(6), 525–530. https://doi.org/10.1089/tmj.2008.0152

Gogia, S. B., Maeder, A., Mars, M., Hartvigsen, G., Basu, A., & Abbott, P. (2016). Unintended consequences of tele health and their possible solutions. Contribution of the IMIA Working Group on Telehealth. *Yearbook of Medical Informatics, 1*, 41-46. doi:10.15265/IY-2016-012

Hampshire, K., Porter, G., Mariwah, S., Munthali, A., Robson, E., Owusu, S. A., Abane, A., & Milner, J. (2017). Who bears the cost of "informal health"? Health-workers' mobile phone practices and associated political-moral economies of care in Ghana and Malawi. *Health Policy & Planning, 32*(1), 34-42. https://doi.org/10.1093/heapol/czw095

Hawker, S., Payne, S., Kerr, C., Hardey, M., & Powell, J. (2002). Appraising the evidence: reviewing disparate data systematically. *Qualitative Health Research, 12*(9), 1284–1299. https://doi.org/10.1177/1049732302238251

Holder-Niles, F., Haynes, L., D'Couto, H., Hehn, R. S., Graham, D. A., Wu, A. C., & Cox, J. E. (2017). Coordinated asthma program improves asthma outcomes in high-risk children. *Clinical Pediatrics, 56*(10), 934–941. https://doi.org/10.1177/0009922817705186.

Holgate, T. S. (2018). A brief history of asthma and its mechanisms to modern concepts of disease pathogenesis. *Journal Allergy Asthma Immunology Research, 2*(3), 165–171. https://doi.org/10.4168/aair.2010.2.3.165

Iyer, S. (2019). Telemedicine stands to offer new horizons to the healthcare solutions landscape. *Global Market Insights.* https://www.mpo-mag.com/contents/view_online- exclusives.

Jayasinghe, D., Crowder, R. M., & Wills, G. (2016). Model for the adoption of telemedicine in Sri Lanka. *SAGE Open.* https://doi.org/10.1177/2158244016668565

Johansson, A. M., Lindberg, I., & Söderberg, S. (2014). Patients' experiences with specialist care via video consultation in primary healthcare in rural areas. *International Journal of Telemedicine and Applications, 9.* https://dl.acm.org/doi/pdf/10.1155/2014/143824

Johansson, A. M., Söderberg, S., & Lindberg, I. (2014). Views of residents of rural areas on accessibility to specialist care through videoconference. *Technology and Health Care, 22*(1), 55-147. https://doi.org/10.3233/THC-140776

John, J., Baek, J., Roh, T., Cabrera-Conner, L., & Carrillo, G. (2017). Regional disparity in asthma prevalence and distribution of asthma education programs in Texas. *Journal of Environmental and Public Health, 2020,* 1–11. https://doi.org/10.1155/2020/9498124

Jong, J. A., Mendez, I. B., & Jong, R. (2019). Enhancing access to care in northern rural communities via telehealth. *International Journal of Circumpolar Health, 78*(2). https://doi.org/10.1080/22423982.2018.1554174

Kennedy, S., Bailey, R., Jaffee, K., Markus, A., Gerstein, M., Stevens, D. M., Lesch, J. K., Malveaux, F. J., & Mitchell, H. (2017). Effectiveness of evidence-based asthma interventions. *Pediatrics, 139.* https://doi.org/10.1542/peds.2016-4221

Kercsmar, C. M., Beck, A. F., Sauers-Ford, H., Simmons, J., Wiener, B., Crosby, L., Wade- Murphy, S., list up to 20 athours Mansour, M. (2017). Association of an asthma improvement collaborative with health care utilization in medicaid-insured pediatric patients in an urban community. *JAMA Pediatrics, 171*(11), 1072–80. 10.1001/jamapediatrics.2017.2600

Kim, T., & Zuckerman, E. J. (2019) Realizing the potential of telemedicine in global health. *Journal of Global Health, 9*(2). https://doi.org/10.7189/jogh.09.020307

Kim, Y., & Pirritano, M. (2019, November). Disparities in health service utilization for asthma: Lower outpatient visits but higher admissions and ED visits among African American children in Los Angeles. In *APHA's 2019 Annual Meeting and Expo (November 2–6). American Public Health Association.*

Koivunen, M., & Saranto, K. (2018). Nursing professionals' experiences of the facilitators and barriers to the use of telehealth applications: A systematic review of qualitative studies. *Scandinavian Journal of Caring Science, 32*(1), 24-44.

Lagerveld, S. E., Bultmann, U., Franche, R. L., van Dijk, F. J., Vlasveld, M. C., van der Feltz- Cornelis, C. M., Bruinvels, D. J., Huijs, J. J., Blonk, R. W., van der Klink, J. J., & Nieuwenhuijsen, K. (2010). Factors associated with work participation and work functioning in depressed workers: a systematic review. *Journal of Occupational Rehabilitation, 20*(3), 275–292.

Leath, B. A., Dunn, L. W., Alsobrook, A., & Darden, M. L. (2018). enhancing rural population health care access and outcomes through the telehealth eco-system model. *Online Journal of Public Health Informatics, 10*(2). https://doi.org/10.5210/ojphi. v10i2.9311

Mammen, R. J., Schoonmaker, D. J., Java J. M. S., Halterman, J., Berliant, N. M, & Crowley, A. (2020). Going mobile with primary care: Smart phone telemedicine for asthma management in young urban adults (Team). *Journal of Asthma, 28*(10). 1273-1277 https://doi.org/10.1080/02770903.2020.183041

Mammen, R. J., Java, J. J., Halterman, J., Berliant, N. M., Crowley, A., Sean, F. M., Reznik, M., Feldman, J. M., Schoonmaker, J. D., & Arcoleo, K. (2019). Development and preliminary results of an Electronic Medical Record (EMR)-integrated smartphone telemedicine program to deliver asthma care remotely. *Journal of Telemedicine and Telecare, 0*(0) 1–14. DOI: 10.1177/1357633X19870025

McElroy, J. A., Day, T. M., & Becevic, M. (2020). The influence of telehealth for better health across communities. *Preventing Chronic Disease, 17*, 1–6. http://dx.doi.org/10.5888/pcd17.200254

McHugh, M. L. (2014). Interrater reliability: The kappa statistic. *Biochemia Medica, 22*(3) 276–282. https://www.ncbi.nlm.nih.gov/pmc/articles/PMC3900052/

McLean, S., Chandler, D., Nurmatov, U., Liu, J., Pagliari, C., Car, J., & Sheikh, A. (2011). Telehealthcare for asthma: A Cochrane review. *CMAJ, 183*(11), E733-E742. 10.1503/cmaj.101146

Miller, J (2019). Death from preventable causes more common in rural vs. urban U.S. *Healio Primary Care Oncology.* Retrieved from www.healio/journal.com

Mistry, H. (2012). Systematic review of studies of the cost-effectiveness of telemedicine and telecare. Changes in the economic evidence over twenty years. *Journal of Telemedicine and Telecare, 18*(1). https://doi.org/10.1258%2Fjtt.2011.110505

Moher, D., Liberati, A., Tetzlaff, J., & Altman, D. G. (2009). Preferred reporting items for systematic reviews and meta-analyses: The PRISMA statement. *Annals of Internal Medicine, 151*(4), 264-269.

Mrkobrada, M., Thiessen-Philbrook, H., Haynes, R. B., Iansavichus, A. V., Rehman, F., & Garg, A. X. (2008). Need for quality improvement in renal systematic reviews. *CJASN, 3*(4), 1102-1114. 10.2215/CJN.04401007.

Naar, S., Ellis, D., Cunningham, P., Pennar, A.L., Lam, P., Brownstein, N.C., & Bruzzese, J. (2018). Comprehensive community-based intervention and asthma outcomes in African American adolescents. *Pediatrics, 142*(4). 10.1542/peds.2017-3737

Nesbitt, T. S. (2012). The evolution of telehealth: Where have we been and where are we going? In Tracy A. Lustig (Ed.), *The role of telehealth in an evolving health care environment: Workshop summary* (pp. 11–15). National Academies Press. https://doi.org/10.17226/ 13466.

Nunes, C., Pereira, A. M., & Morais-Almeida, M., (2017). Asthma costs and social impact. *Asthma Research and Practice, 3.* https://doi.org/10.1186/s40733-016-0029-3

Nurmagambetov, T., Kuwahara, R., & Garbe, P. (2018). The economic burden of asthma in the United States, 2008-2013. *Annals of the American Thoracic Society, 15*(3), 348-356. https://doi.org/10.1513/AnnalsATS.201703-259OC

Perry, T.T., Halterman, J.S., Brown, R.H., Luo, C., Randle, S.M., Hunter, C.R., & Rettiganti, M. (2018). Results of an asthma education program delivered via telemedicine in rural schools. *Annals of Allergy, Asthma, & Immunology, 120*(4), 401-408. https://doi.org/10.1016/j.anai.2018.02.013

Perry, T.T. & Turner, T.H. (2019). School-based telemedicine for asthma management. *Journal of Allergy and Clinical Immunology: In Practice, 7*(8), 2524-2532. https://doi.org/10.1016/j.jaip.2019.08.009

Pierce, R. P., & Stevermer, J. J. (2020). Disparities in use of telehealth at the onset of the COVID-19 public health emergency. *Journal of Telemedicine and Telecare*, 1357633X20963893. Advance online publication. https://doi.org/10.1177/1357633X20963893.

Punch, K. F. (2013). *Introduction to social research: Quantitative and qualitative approaches.* Thousand Oaks, CA: Sage Publications

Quirt, J., Hildebrand, K. J., Mazza, J., Noya, F., & Kim, H. (2018). Asthma. *Allergy, Asthma & Clinical Immunology, 14*(2), 16–30. https://doi.org/10.1186/s13223-018-0279-0

Rapp, K. I., Jack, L., Wilson, C., Hayes, S. C., Post, R., McKnight, E., & Malveaux, F. (2018). Improving asthma-related outcomes among children participating in the head-off environmental asthma in Louisiana (HEAL), Phase II Study. *Health Promotion Practice, 19*(2), 233–239. https://doi.org/10.1177/1524839917740126

Rasulnia, M., Burton, S. B., Ginter, R. P., Wang, Y. T., Pleasants A. R., Green, L. C, & Lugogo, N. (2018). Assessing the impact of a remote digital coaching engagement program on patient-reported outcomes in asthma. *Journal of Asthma, 55*(7).795-800. https://doi.org/10.1080/02770903.2017.1362430

Rubin, H. J., & Rubin, I. S. (2012). *Qualitative interviewing: The art of hearing data* (3rd ed.). Thousand Oaks, CA: Sage Publications.

Sabesan, S., Senko, C., Schmidt, A., Joshi, A., Pandey, R., Ryan, C. A., Lyle, M., Rainey, N., Varma, S., Otty, Z., Ansari, Z., Vaughan, K., Vangaveti, V., Black, J., & Brown, A. (2018). Enhancing chemotherapy capabilities in rural hospitals: Implementation of a telechemotherapy model (QReCS) in North Queensland, Australia. *Journal of Oncology Practice, 14*(7), e429-e437. https://doi.org/10.1200/JOP.18.00110

Sadreameli, S. C., Riekert, K. A., Matsui, E. C., Rand, C. S., & Eakin, M. N. (2018). Family caregiver marginalization is associated with decreased primary and subspecialty asthma care in Head Start children. *Academic Pediatrics, 18*(8), 905-911. https://doi.org/10.1016/j.acap.2018.04.135

Schwamm, L. H., Chumbler, N., Brown, E., Fonarow, G. C., Berube, D., Nystrom, K., Suter, R., Zavala, M., Polsky, D., Radhakrishnan, K., Lacktman, N., Horton, K., Malcarney, M., Halamka, J., & Tiner, A. C. (2017). Recommendations for the implementation of telehealth in cardiovascular and stroke care: A policy statement from the American Heart Association. *Circulation, 135*(7). https://doi.org/ 10.1161/ cir.0000000000000475

Taylor, L., Waller, M., & Portnoy, J. (2019). Telemedicine for allergy services to rural communities. *Journal of Allergy and Clinical Immunology: In Practice, 7*(8),2554- 2559. https://doi.org/10.1016/j.jaip.2019.06.012

To, T., Stanojevic, S., Moores, G., Garshon, A. S., Bateman, E. D., Cruz, A., & Boulet, L.space P. (2012). Global asthma prevalence in adults: Findings from the cross-sectional world health survey. *BMC Public Health, 12*, 1–8. https://doi.org/10.1186/1471-2458-12-204

Totten, M. A., McDonagh, S. M., & Wagner, H. S. (2020). The evidence bases for telehealth: reassurance in the face of rapid expansion during the COVID-19 pandemic. *Agency for*

Healthcare Research and Quality. https://doi.org/10.23970/ AHRQEPCCOVID TELEHEALTH.

Trivedi, M., Fung, V., Kharbanda, E. O., Larkin, E. K., Butler, M. G., Horan, K., Lieu, T. A., & Wu, A. C. (2018). Racial disparities in family-provider interactions for pediatric asthma care. *Journal of Asthma, 55*(4), 424-429.

Turyk, M., Banda, E., Chisum, G., Weems, D. Jr, Liu. Y., Damitz, M., Williams, R., & Persky, V. (2013). A multifaceted community-based asthma intervention in Chicago: Effects of trigger reduction and self-management education on asthma morbidity. *Journal of Asthma, 50*(7), 729–736. https://doi.org/1 0.3109/02770903.2013.796971

Van Veen, T., Binz, S., Muminovic, M., Chaudhry, K., Rose, K., Calo, S., Rammal, J. A., France, J., & Miller, J. B. (2019). Potential of mobile health technology to reduce health disparities in underserved communities. *Western Journal of Emergency Medicine, 20*(5), 799–802. https://doi.org/10.5811/ westjem.2019.6.41911

Walter, J. M., & Holtzman, J. M. (2005). A centennial history of research on asthma pathogenesis. *American Journal of Respiratory Cell and Molecular Biology, 32*(6), 483–489. https:// doi.org/10.1165/rcmb.F300

Wainwright, C. & Wootton, R. (2003). A review of telemedicine and asthma. *Disease Management and Health Outcomes, 11*, 557–563. https://doi.org/10.2165/00115677- 200311090-0000

Wootton, R., A, Geissbuhler, A., B, Jethwani, J., C, Kovarik, C., D, Person, D. A., E., Vladzymyrskyy, A., F., Zanaboni, F., A., & Zolfo, M. (2012). Long-running telemedicine networks delivering humanitarian services: Experience, performance, and scientific output. *Bulletin of the World Health Organization, 90*, 341-347D. https://doi.org/10.2471/BLT.11.099143

World Health Organization. (2015). Telehealth. https://www.who. int/gho/goe/telehealth/en/

World Health Organization. (2021). Telehealth. https://www.who.int/gho/goe/telehealth/en/

Zhao, J., Zhai, Y., Zhu, W., & Sun, D. (2015). Effectiveness of telemedicine for controlling asthma symptoms: A systematic review and meta-analysis. *Telemedicine Journal and e-Health: The Official Journal of the American Telemedicine Association, 21*(6), 484-92. https://doi.org/10.1089/tmj.2014.011

APPENDICES

Appendix A
Coding Guidelines

1. Articles selected using the search strategy should be read completely to ensure that it meets all inclusion criteria.
2. Inclusion Criteria
   i. Date: Literature published between January 1, 2013, through May 31, 2021
   ii. Language: English
   iii. Type of publication: Peer-reviewed
   iv. Study design: randomized controlled trials, interventional trials, trials that are not strictly randomized, and non-randomized trials, such as observational, and case studies
   v. Studies must have adults aged 18-55 years old with asthma diagnosis, has at least one asthma intervention through telemedicine outcome endpoint
3. Exclusion Criteria
   i. Articles are not editorials, commentaries, opinion papers, systematic reviews, or letters to the editor will not be included
   ii. Studies with only telemedicine intervention with asthma care either through smart phone interface, video conferencing, emailing communication and simultaneous usual care (face to face) visit.
   iii. Studies that only have participants residing in large metropolitans and urban cities areas.

4. After completing full review of each article, determine whether the publication is still eligible.
   i. If it is, identify if there are any companion article to search and evaluate.
   ii. If no, document the reason for not including the study.
5. Each rater should complete the coding sheet for each article reviewed.
   i. A table for each study will be completed with rater 1 and rater 2 information for all inclusion and exclusion criteria and calculations completed
   ii. Calculate the kappa coefficient
6. After completing the coding, tbe raters should discuss the articles that had discrepancies between the raters.
   i. Discuss the concerns
   ii. Review the articles again
   iii. Do not change the initial answers
   iv. Complete a second version of the coding table for the articles that were inconsistent
   v. If inconsistencies persist, a new line for coding should be determined and included
7. After completing the reconciled articles, the author should fill out the final data extraction tables.
8. Note issues and concerns that may cause a hinder in coming to an agreement.

Appendix B

Interpretation of Cohen's Kappa

κ value	Agreement
<0	Less than chance agreement
0.01–0.20	Slight agreement
0.21–0.40	Fair agreement
0.41–0.60	Moderate agreement
0.61–0.80	Substantial agreement
0.81–0.99	Almost perfect agreement

Note: Adapted from https://www.ncbi.nlm.gov/pmc/articles/PMC 3900052/

Appendix C
Selection of the Five Studies to Include for Review According to the Two Raters

Study Title	Is the study peer-reviewed?	Is the study in English?	Does the publication date fall within the period of January 1, 2013, to May 31, 2021?	Was the telemedicine outcome measured/reported?	Was the study type a trial, observational study, or case study?	Are exclusion criteria absent? The study was not a theoretical paper, opinion paper, letter to the editor, a commentary, systematic review, or metanalysis?	Are the exclusion criteria absent? The study was not on patients with primary diagnoses not asthma, did not receive telemedicine interventions?. Participants ages not outside of range of 18 to 55 years? Participants not residents outside urban or metropolitan areas?	Agreement between the reviewers regarding selection criteria
Going mobile with primary care: Smart phone telemedicine for asthma management in young urban adults (Team)	Y/Y	Y/Y	Y/Y	Y/Y	Y/Y	Y/Y	Y/Y	7 of 7
Assessing the impact of a remote digital Coaching engagement program on patient-reported outcomes in asthma.	Y/Y	Y/Y	Y/Y	Y/Y	Y/Y	Y/Y	Y/Y	7 of 7

The "physician on call patient engagement trail" (POPET): measuring the impact of a mobile patient engagement application on health outcomes and quality of life in allergic rhinitis and asthma patients	Y/Y	Y/Y	Y/Y	Y/Y	Y/Y	Y/Y	7 of 7
Development and Preliminary results of an Electronic Medical Record (EMR)-integrated smartphone telemedicine program to deliver asthma care remotely	Y/Y	Y/Y	Y/Y	Y/Y	Y/Y	Y/Y	7 of 7
Long-term outcomes on internet-based self-management support in adult asthma:	Y/Y	Y/Y	Y/Y	Y/Y	Y/Y	Y/Y	7 of 7

Note: Data are given as Rater 1 / Rater 2.

Appendix D

Selection of the Six Studies to Exclude from Review According to the Two Raters

Study Title	Is the study peer-reviewed?	Is the study in English?	Does the publication date fall within the period of January 1, 2013, to May 31, 2021?	Was the telemedicine outcome measured/reported?	Was the study type a trial, observational study, or case study?	Are exclusion criteria absent? The study was not a theoretical paper, opinion paper, letter to the editor, a commentary, systematic review, or metanalysis?	Are the exclusion criteria absent? The study was not on patients with primary diagnoses not asthma, did not receive telemedicine interventions?. Participants ages not outside of range of 18 to 55 years? Participants not residents outside urban or metropolitan areas?	Agreement between the reviewers regarding selection criteria
The active patient role and asthma outcomes in the underserved rural communities	Y/Y	Y/Y	Y/Y	N/N	Y/Y	N/N	Y/Y	5 of 7
Remote monitoring of inhaled bronchodilator use and weekly feedback about asthma management.	Y/Y	Y/Y	Y/Y	N/N	Y/Y	N/N	N/N	4 of 7

Description								
Evaluation of asthma medication adherence rates and strategies to improve adherence in the underserved population at a federally qualified health center	Y/Y	Y/Y	Y/Y	N/N	Y/Y	N/N	N/N	4 of 7
Effectiveness of population health management using the Propeller Health asthma platform:	Y/Y	Y/Y	Y/Y	Y/Y	Y/Y	N/N	N/N	5 of 7
The effective web-based asthma self-management system, asthma portal (MAP)	Y/	Y/	Y/Y	Y/Y	Y/Y	N/N	N/N	5 of 7
A patient-centered mobile health system that supports asthma self-management (BREATHE).	Y/Y	Y/Y	Y/Y	N/N	Y/Y	N/N	N/N	4 of 7

Note: Data are given as Rater 1 / Rater 2.

Appendix E
Data Analysis Table for the Five Articles in the Systematic Review

Study Title	Year Published	Authors	Journal	Type of Study/Design	Location	Objective	Sample Population	Sample Size	Results/Outcomes	Biases/Limitations	Funded? (Yes/No)	Study Duration
Going mobile with primary care: Smartphone telemedicine for asthma management in young urban adults (Team)	2020	Mammen RJ, Schoonmaker JD, Hallerwon J, Berliant MJ, Crowley A,	Journal of Asthma	Mixed Method Randomized Trail	New York. USA	Deliver asthma care remotely	Adults aged 18-44 years with persistent chronically uncontrolled asthma	33	Reduced asthma symptoms and improved quality of life	Research related incentive/High frequency follow up visits	Not	3- 6 months.
Assessing the impact of a remote digital Coaching engagement program on patient-reported outcomes in asthma.	2018	Rasulnia M, Burton SB, Ginter PR, Wang YT, Alton P, et al	Journal of Asthma	Prospective Cohort Studies	North Carolina, USA	Examine impact of remote digital coaching program on asthma control and patient experience	>18 years old with current uncontrolled asthma noted by albuterol use >2 times weekly or requiring systematic corticosteroids	40	Decreased acute asthma worsening symptoms. Improved asthma medication compliance. Successful tobacco cessation	Short study periods Small sample size 20% drop-out rate Lack of cost analysis Study sample predominantly female	Funded	3 months

The "physician on call patient engagement trial" (POPET): measuring the impact of a mobile patient engagement application on health outcomes and quality of life in allergic rhinitis and asthma patients	2015	Cingi C, Yorgancioglu A, Cingi CC, Oguzulgen K, Muluk NB, et al	International Forum of Allergy & Rhinology	Prospective Randomized controlled double-blinded trail	Turkey	Investigated the impact of a mobile patient engagement application on health outcomes and quality of life in allergic rhinitis (AR) and asthma patients	Adults aged 21-50 years with diagnosis of mild to severe persistent asthma or diagnosis of persistent allergic rhinitis for at least 2 years, and smartphone users for at least six months	327	Significant statistical improvement in satisfaction with allergy and asthma symptoms	High attrition rate in controlled group	Not	3 months

95

Title	Year	Authors	Journal	Design	Location	Aim	Population	N	Results	Limitations	Funded	Duration
Development and Preliminary results of an Electronic Medical Record (EMR)-integrated smartphone telemedicine program to deliver asthma care remotely.	2019	Mammen JR, Java JJ, Halterman J, Berliant NM, Crowley A, et al	Journal of Telemedicine and Telecare	Contextually grounded intervention development approach	New York, UAS	Clinically integrate smartphone-telemedicine program in care of adults with asthma	Adults aged 18-40 with current diagnosis of Asthma. Speaks English and have a smartphone.	7	Improved asthma control Improved quality of life Improved patient satisfaction	Small sample size. Participants younger, minority, lower socioeconomic status, lower health literacy, Interventions by single provider	Funded	3 months
Long-Term outcomes on internet-Based Self-Management Support in Adults Asthma	2013	Gaalen JL, Beerthuizen T, Meer V, Reisen P, Redelikheaid GW, Snoeck-Stroband JW, et al	Journal of Medical Internet Research	Randomized Controlled Trial	Leiden, Netherlands	To assess the long-term effects of providing internet-based self-management care compared to usual care	Adults 18-50 years	200	Significant improvement in asthma symptom control and asthma-related quality of life.	Low response rate Differences of improved asthma symptoms and quality of life for IG (Internet group) and UC (Usual care-face to face), not significantly great	Not	2-3 years

Printed in the United States
by Baker & Taylor Publisher Services